READY-SET-MARKET!

By
Andrea T. Eliscu

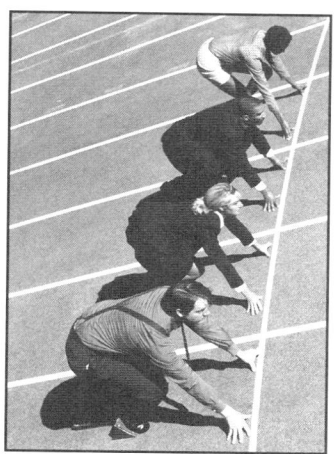

Published by:
Medical Group Management Association
104 Inverness Terrace East
Englewood CO 80112
(888) 608-5601
Web site: http://www.mgma.com

Medical Group Management Association (MGMA) publications are intended to provide current and accurate information and are designed to assist readers in becoming more familiar with the subject matter covered. Such publications are distributed with the understanding that MGMA does not render any legal, accounting or other professional advice that may be construed as specifically applicable to individual situations. No representations or warranties are made concerning the application of legal or other principles discussed by the author to any specific factual situation, nor is any prediction made concerning how any particular judge, government official or other person will interpret or apply such principles. Specific factual situations should be discussed with professional advisors.

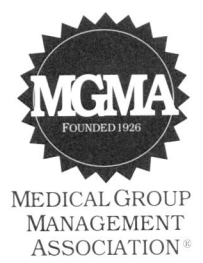

MEDICAL GROUP
MANAGEMENT
ASSOCIATION®

Acknowledgments

It is with sincere appreciation that I would like to recognize the clients, colleagues and friends who have contributed to this book. Writing this book has been an intense experience and one that has been a result of teaming and partnering during my 33 years in the health care industry.

I thank each and every one of you for encouraging me to lead and implement my vision for health care marketing and positioning. Many of you have been mentors and generously shared your knowledge with me.

This book is dedicated to my husband, Edward H. Eliscu, MD, who is a warrior in my eyes.

I would also like to say thank you to Mary Scott, Richard J. Walsh, Lori Johnson, John Bruns, Barbara Ann Blue, Dan Frankel, Bob Kodzis, David Cassidy, Jay Pearce, Hedrick Rivero, MD, Robert Westergan, MD, Becky Cherney, Christopher Rolle and Natalie Roussman for sharing their marketing insights.

In addition, my appreciation goes to Cynthia Kiyotake, MS, Director of the MGMA Library Resource Center, and to Alys Novak, MGMA Acquisition Editor, for their support during the book's editorial stage, as well as to the production team of Network Graphics, Brian Novak and Heather McHugh.

Table of Contents

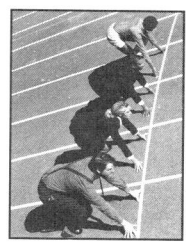

Introduction

Grass Roots Marketing in a New Millennium

"Be it furniture, clothes or health care, many industries today are marketing nothing more than commodities—no more, no less. What will make the difference in the long run is the care and feeding of customers."

— Michael and Timothy Mescon,
How to Win Customers and Keep Them for Life

Although literally hundreds of texts have been written about how to market a medical practice, when it comes right down to it, it's not all that complicated. Or, as one colleague puts it, it's not brain surgery.

In the new millennium—just as in the past—it pretty much can be boiled down to one thing. **Customer service.**

In today's business environment—*and make no mistake about it, medicine today **is** a business*—all the marketing in the world won't make you succeed if you fail to remember your customers are your number one priority. Quite simply, if you don't keep them happy, they'll find someone who will.

Retailers know it. Restaurateurs know it. Hotel managers, in particular, know it. Why don't health care providers understand it?

Many, of course, do. They're the smart ones—usually, the ones whose practices are **successful.** They're the ones who hire competent people, train those people well and pay a motivating wage. They're the ones who know what matters most to their patients—because they ask—and respond positively to what they're told.

Smart practices also know that today's customers **expect** quality care—even demand it. And, they expect more. Research shows that close to 70 percent of customers don't go back to a business due to the indifferent or negative attitude of the owner, manager or an employee. Even simple body language may be enough to create the wrong impression.

In fact, studies also show verbal communications (words) account for only about 10 percent of the total message we convey. Another 40 percent is imparted by voice tone, while fully half of all communication occurs through body language.

In addition, many businesses never know why dissatisfied customers leave, because most don't complain. They simply "vote with their feet"—by walking out the door and into that of a competitor down the street.

What can you do to make your practice one of the ones that succeeds?

The simple answer is to be proactive. Make good customer relations programs an integral part of your practice every day, in every way, in every message you send to your customers—whether patients, employers, referrers, managed care companies or others.

For example, before you open your door each morning, make sure your staff is prepared, your office is well kept and your policies are clearly written. Make sure systems are in place to make your patients feel not just welcome, but valued. And make sure each person in your office knows and shares your philosophy.

In other words, make customer service the grass roots (defined as "what is basic, fundamental") of your marketing in the new millennium.

Of course, there's more to it than that. I'm not suggesting that you should rely on customer service as your only marketing tool. I'm simply saying that it is the vital element necessary to help you build a strong foundation for marketing success over time. (Chapter 2 explores this issue further.)

As we move into the next millennium, it's obvious that health care is being redesigned as a result of social and political forces. These include:
- Health care is becoming more bureaucratic;
- Consumers play a greater, more assertive role in decision-making;
- Third-party payers continue to increase their demands on hospitals and physicians;
- Government regulations continue to increase and intrude in group practice operations at an escalated rate;

- Medicare and Medicaid continue to lower reimbursements;
- There are more capitated managed care contracts;
- The cost of pharmaceuticals continues to increase;
- Practices have to absorb costs associated with Y2K compliance as they prepare for the next century; and
- Medical excellence and patient service continue to be a focal point of competition.

Ultimately, you can enhance your chances of survival and control your destiny as a free enterprise if you strive to give your customers:

- Service excellence—every day, in every way;
- Community involvement;
- Cost containment;
- Responsible, educated, dedicated and empowered leadership; and
- Academic achievement on a continuous basis for physicians and staff.

The purpose of this book is to provide a practical, quick and easy "how-to" guide for medical group marketing. I hope it will open the door to communications that will help you position for success by understanding the importance of marketing, building the right foundation for it, and preparing the vital tools you need for success.

One way to learn is by example. Emulate others who have a reputation for exemplary customer service and a record of success in the marketplace. Throughout the book, such examples will be presented, along with case studies and other sample programs I hope you will find useful.

The first example, in the following chapter, was provided by John Bruns, general manager of a prestigious four-star hotel chain known around the world as a symbol of top quality and unequaled service. I hope you find it, as well as the other examples throughout the book, interesting and informative. My goal is to have you take something away from each of them that will help you make your marketing program more successful.

Figure Introduction-a

Customer-service motivational techniques

Wonder how you can motivate your employees? Study the example of the Daytona International Speedway, cited by John Koenig, business columnist for the *"Orlando Sentinel's Central Florida Business"* section (February 8-14, 1999). Reprinted with permission.

Speedway workers get a theme song for customer-service track

Daytona Beach — Between races at the 1999 Daytona International Speedway, the loudspeakers around the track blared out the old Beach Boys' hit "Good Vibrations."

Race fans, no doubt, thought the song was for them. It wasn't, at least not directly.

The primary target was the people working at the track. It was to remind them of the lessons they had been taught on providing good customer service and to ask themselves, "Am I sending out good vibrations?"

Like a lot of businesses, Daytona International Speedway has been focusing more attention lately on improving customer service.

You might think the track would not need to do that. After all, its premiere event, the Daytona 500, is the most-watched motor-sports event in the country—on television and in person. Some 200,000 people packed the grandstand and infield at this year's race.

But those fans arrived with high expectations, having spent a minimum of $65 for a ticket and having traveled an average of 200 miles to get there. A great race is only part of what they wanted from their time at the speedway.

"If the rest of the experience is disappointing to them, then we, like any other business, are in danger of losing them," says John Graham, president of the Speedway. A discourteous parking lot attendant or a surly security guard could cause a customer never to come back again.

So whom did the track rely on to provide great customer service? Mainly, part-timers—people who worked there only a few days of the year. The speedway hired 2,000 workers to work just during the Daytona 500.

The track added customer service training for its part-time employees four years ago. In 1998, for the Pepsi 400 race, it decided to try something different.

Working through Daytona Beach Community College's Center for Business, it brought in training consultant Donna M. Long of Kissimmee, Florida. Long has been experimenting with music as a way to reinforce training messages.

She came up with the idea of building the track's customer-service program around the song "Good Vibrations." And she developed a customer service acronym on the word VIBES. At the speedway, it stands for: VIPs (all fans), Immediate service, Body language, Eye contact and Smiles.

Among the things she talked about during a two-hour training session with about 50 track workers was the importance of body language in conveying the right impression to customers. She said that only 10 percent of all communication occurs through words, that 40 percent occurs through voice tone and 50 percent through body language.

For much of the session, Long showed pictures of common interactions between customers and workers at the track and led discussions on how workers might handle those situations. For instance, how should an employee respond if a fan tries to climb over a fence to a restricted area? By explaining why the area is restricted, Long said.

An hour is not much time to turn a novice employee into a customer-service expert. But that's where the music came in. During the session, Long played the Beach Boys' song several times. When the employees heard the song on race day, they were reminded how important it was to send "Good Vibrations" out to the customers.

Am I suggesting that you start blaring "Good Vibrations" throughout your office? Of course not. I'm simply saying, take this example and try to apply it to your situation. Learn from the success of others.

Figure Introduction-b

One patient's experience

My 72-year-old father, a diabetic, appeared as scheduled at the local medical center for an 8:30 a.m. fasting blood test. The front desk worker loudly informed him that she didn't have a record of his appointment and that the first time he could be seen was at 11:30 a.m. that same day. When he explained that he was a diabetic and really shouldn't wait that long to eat, she told him, that was too bad. No one could see him any sooner. Not wanting to argue but determined not to go without his breakfast, he simply walked away. As he reached the door, the worker shouted, "Hey, you can't leave." My father replied, "Like hell I can't." and continued out the door. He got a new doctor, and so did I!

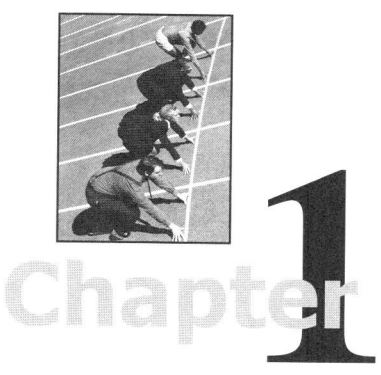

Chapter 1

READY: How to Keep Your Customers Coming Back

"If you would hit the mark, you must aim a little above it; every arrow that flies feels the attraction of the earth."

—Henry Wadsworth Longfellow

Most of you recognize that reimbursement is one major focus in the health care industry right now. Obviously, an issue that hits everyone's style of living is important. However, you may not be aware of the other big, consistent—very topical—issue: customer service. In the long term, I believe this issue is just as important as any other to the success of your practice.

In other industries, customer service has high priority. For example, when I observed the relationship between Richard Harris and the Ritz-Carlton in Cleveland, I saw many connections between the hourly workers hired to work in the hospitality industry and the workers that we hire in health care. I asked the hotel's manager to discuss how his hotel chain had become the icon for service in the hotel industry. I asked him how he found employees with the core values to meet the hotel's mission statement. I also asked him how he motivates new hires and young staff people to perform their best during the hours on the job.

A hospitality professional with more than 25 years experience, John F. Bruns is General Manager of the Ritz-Carlton, Cleveland. He also served as vice president of development for Renaissance Hotels International and as general manager of the Stouffer Renaissance Chicago hotel. Other experience includes general manager of the Stouffer Nashville Hotel and management positions with Westin Hotels and Resorts in San Francisco, Seattle, Detroit, Cincinnati and Chicago.

The following discussion features Bruns' perspective from the hotel industry. I believe you will see a connection between his perspective and your role as leadership in your health care organization or group practice.

Want a reputation for excellent customer service?
Here's how to achieve it.

Hire the best people you can. Engage those people in your philosophy and values toward service. Train and motivate them, recognize and reward them. Grow your business so they are challenged and learn from new experiences. Finally, improve their quality of life by paying them more to take on increased responsibility and thus, make a larger contribution to your organization.

Easy to say. Tough to do.

Customer service is that "moment of truth," that moment of interaction between two people that defines your organization. If the interaction is positive, the moment adds to your reputation. If the moment takes on negative tones, your reputation is eroded. If the moment of truth is neutral—neither positive nor negative—there is no change in your reputation in the mind of your customer.

So who are your customers, and how do you ensure that these "moments of truth" are positive?

In the hotel business, the three primary customers a manager serves are the guest, the owner and the employee. Although it is a challenge, balancing the needs of these constituent groups is the key to success. Why? The simple answer: A decision in favor of one often negatively impacts the other two.

For instance, let's look at what the owners want. They want more cash flow to invest in the physical product or to return to the shareholders. Obviously, squeezing profits through cutting quality may have a short-term benefit. However, it may produce the long-term consequences of poor employee morale and disappointed guests.

What about employees? They want better working conditions, higher pay and shorter hours. A decision in favor of the employees will definitely impact owner cash flow.

And, consider the guests. What do they want? Lower rates, faster service, better and cleaner accommodations—all imposing more cost on the owners and more effort on the employees.

It's apparent that balancing your decisions and actions to meet the needs of customers cannot be done in a vacuum. It has to be based on the philosophy and values of the organization.

Most organizations express their values and philosophy in their mission statements, which typically, define the purpose of the organization. The shortest mission statement might be "to attract and maintain customers." Again, if the customers are hotel guests, employees and owners, then the purpose is to attract and maintain all of them. The simplicity of this mission statement adds to its value.

For instance, any and all decisions, actions and behaviors of the organization must be defensible when measured against the necessity to balance the needs of all customers: guest, owner or an employee. Thus, values and philosophies, when expressed in the form of a mission statement guide the behaviors of the organization and form the cornerstone of the reputation of the organization.

While a mission statement may be held up to define a practice's values and philosophy, the actions and behaviors of its people speak louder than words. How, then, does the organization align people's behavior with the philosophy and create a reputation for great customer service? It starts with your employee process.

The employee process can be broken down into six steps:
- Recruiting;
- Selection;
- Hiring;
- Orientation;
- Skill training; and
- Certification.

During each of these steps, your practice has the opportunity to reinforce your beliefs, values and philosophy. In fact, your employment process is the foundation for building a reputation for great customer service. Let's walk through these steps.

Recruiting

The ability to attract prospective employees to your hospital or group practice is based on the perception of your business as a place to work. Employment advertising, direct participation in job fairs, and importantly, word-of-mouth and referrals of current employees form the perception of your work environment.

Talent attracts talent, and in a large group practice, it obviously makes sense to invest in a dynamic, resourceful, and trustworthy leader in human resources. In a small group, this may be the CEO. Nevertheless, the ability to communicate the mission enthusiastically, along with the work environment, the compensation and the career opportunities, will have a major impact on the impression your organization makes on an applicant.

Selection

What talent is required to be successful in a position? Starting with a job description, there may be certain skills that are required and some skills that are "nice to have." Highly focused companies, such as the Ritz-Carlton Hotel Company (RCHC), have taken the selection of talent from an art to a science.

For example, RCHC has profiled the characteristics of highly successful people in every position in the company. Benchmarking the highly successful "control group" against all other workers in that job category defines a range of acceptability for job applicants. Importantly, 85 percent of the individuals tested in or above the range are successful, while 85 percent of the applicants hired below the range fail the organization in the first year.

Obviously, there are no guarantees in selecting people to join the organization, but the point is that there should be a basis of non-discriminatory criteria to improve the chance of success.

Hiring

Hiring an individual is the most important decision made by the organization. Once hired, this person represents the company during and after work. Some helpful hints on hiring:

- Have the applicant interview with many people in the organization: male, female, supervisor, peer. Get perspective.
- Interview the candidate at 7 a.m. one day, 6 p.m. another. Some people are morning people, some are night people.
- Stay in constant contact and check references.
- Shorten your cycle time and don't lose a "hot prospect" to your competitor.
- Look at your employment area—the physical appearance and how people are treated when they apply. Does it attract talent?

Orientation

The Ritz-Carlton believes that orientation is mandatory—no exceptions—prior to the first day on the job. It seems that medical practices should do the same. Successful service companies, such as Disney, Darden Restaurants and Nordstrom, require orientation prior to the employee ever coming in contact with a customer.

Typically, orientations cover work rules, policies, procedures, and key philosophies and values of the organization. Disney, for example, brings new employees to a room filled with posters and memorabilia from the early days of Walt Disney and Mickey Mouse. Once in this room, the new employees take a test! The catch is that all the answers to the test are in the room, and employees are encouraged to help each other. Importantly, new employees leave that day knowing key facts about the beginnings of the company and the importance of teamwork.

Whatever format an organization chooses to employ, mandatory orientation sets the stage for new employees—how they will be treated and how they feel about their new role in the organization. Don't miss this opportunity to demonstrate your practice's commitment to great customer service.

Skill training

Job descriptions, job breakdowns and task analysis all are important components of skill training. But how do these skills lead to great customer service?

Job skill mastery leads to confidence and high self-esteem, both important characteristics of successful service employees. The mastery of job skills is important, but the people skills of the individual are what separate the good employee from the great employee. Certainly, somewhere in your practice's values and philosophy should be a strong statement of the beliefs of how people should take care of people. That "Moment of Truth," the interaction between two human beings, needs to be constantly refined and developed during the period of skill training.

RCHC, for example, has a motto of "Ladies and Gentlemen Serving Ladies and Gentlemen." The motto serves as a standard of behavior founded on the principle of respect for one another. Respect in the workplace leads to trust, teamwork and harmony. Certainly, any organization defined in such terms would be a good place to work and would be a magnet for attracting high potential employees.

Certification

After a period of employment, testing and verification of skills confirm new employees are fully qualified to serve the customers. Such verification should serve to reinforce the values and philosophy of the company as well as measure job skill development. Certification should be fun and should allow employees to express their views on the first few weeks of employment. Sharing information, in an open and honest format, builds trust and respect in the workplace. We're all on the same team, and the certification process, symbolized by a Certificate of Achievement, provides recognition and reward for new employees in their roles as customer service agents.

Now that the organization has attracted talent and invested valuable resources in the employment process, how does the company keep its people and engage them in performance at a high level of service excellence?

Maintaining customers, external (guests) or internal (employees), is the true test of an organization. Many service industries, such as hotels, restaurants and resorts, are plagued with high turnover. In fact, one hotel company is so concerned about employee retention that it is a major portion of all managers' incentive compensation.

The connection between retention and great customer service is consistency. If the organization retains talented people, fully engaged in the skills and value of customer service, then the organization will consistently perform at peak levels.

On the other hand, organizations with high turnover risk poor quality service, the outcome of new employee mistakes and tired employees working extra shifts in "short staff" service situations.

Poor quality service drives external customers away and provides sufficient reason for remaining talented employees (internal customers) to question why they should remain with the organization.

So, how do you keep talent? Here are seven things you can do to create a positive work environment:

1. Train on an on-going basis.

Ritz-Carlton believes training is critical to the retention of talented people. Talented people love to learn and grow. Training provides the opportunity to demonstrate the commitment to customer service, provides additional tools or skills for providing better service and for aligning customer service with personal benefits to the individual. Training reinforces the existing base of knowledge of the employee and expands the base with exposure to new ideas, concepts and methods.

Simply put, when talented people aren't challenged, or if they feel they have stopped learning and growing, they leave you to find and satisfy that need somewhere else!

2. Provide recognition and reward.

What drives your employees to greatness? Chances are it is different things for different people. For some it's money, public recognition or letters of commendation. For others, it may be a pat on the back, a one-on-one thank you, or it may be a letter to their parents!

Quite frequently, employees in the hotel industry are visited by their parents who stay in the hotel. Just imagine how much self-esteem would be deposited to the employee if the manager of the hotel upgraded the accommodations and wrote a personal note to the parents praising their son's or daughter's contributions to the team!

Whatever the basis of recognition and rewards—time and attendance, outstanding service such as "above and beyond the call," lateral service to another employee— the concentration of effort should be consistent and meaningful to the employment group. Think about it. Recognition is critical to your team. As the old saying goes, "What gets rewarded, gets repeated!"

3. Compensate fairly.

Money is another form of recognition. Presumably, the organization has a hierarchy of pay scales based on relative contribution to the business. If not, you may want to start grading jobs by grouping like duties and responsibilities in areas such as customer contact, number of people reporting to the position, education or skill requirements, where the position reports, access to confidential information and, importantly, impact on the medical practice. Once a job tier of grades is established, then a local wage survey of similar and different businesses can be conducted to benchmark local wages.

From experience, an open, honest approach with employees on the job grading and salaries is best, but it takes annual training to reinforce the integrity of the program. During this annual training, you have another opportunity to discuss increases in the scale based on inflation or cost-of-living, as well as to remind employees that the best way to improve their earnings is to take on new responsibility through a promotion.

Clearly, establishing a framework and paying for performance reinforces the objectivity of a compensation program and minimizes claims against the business relative to wage discrimination.

One final thought. Most hourly employees know what their co-workers are making, so open and honest communication goes a long way toward attracting and maintaining talent.

4. Communicate openly and constantly.

Clear communications is the single most powerful tool in motivating people. Here is an example.

A 17-year-old student spends hours working on a history paper on the subject of the Viet Nam war. Presenting his paper to the teacher, he is told, "I'm sorry, I cannot accept your paper. The assignment was for you to write on a war fought on U.S. property."

How does the student feel? Stupid, frustrated, angry and upset are a few words that come to mind. The "moment of truth" between the teacher and the student did not improve their relationship. Rather, it was emotional and had negative tones of anger, disappointment and mistrust.

This entire experience was caused by poor communications. Simply put, if you do not clearly communicate the needs of the organization (good customer service), you are not likely to get what you expect. Clear communications at least improve the chances of getting the desired behavior and outcome from other people. And, when people receive clear communications, which results in desired performance or outcomes, it is a positive motivating experience when recognized and rewarded by peers and supervisors.

5. Commit to career planning.

The fact is, not every employee is set on a career in your industry. Some people are in the job only to support school or some other profession. On the other hand, some members of the team want a career in the health care industry, and their expectations of the job are a concern.

One simple system to meet expectations is to meet with every employee who has worked for the group over a certain period of time, such as one year. Find out what their goals are, what skills need to be acquired to take on more responsibility, how the organization can help—possibly in the form of co-paying tuition costs.

Again, clear communications on what it will take to move ahead is a very positive and motivating session with an employee. It builds expectations also, so be sure to put these in writing and follow up on commitments.

6. Act on employee surveys.

Employee satisfaction is often termed employee morale. Satisfaction and morale are tough to gauge. Certainly, the larger the work group, the more difficult it is to measure, given the exponential interactions between co-workers.

Nevertheless, employee surveys of large and small work groups, when done on a confidential basis by an independent third party, can reveal important trends in the workplace. By knowing the weaknesses and strengths of the work environment, proper action can be taken to address concerns of the employees.

Notwithstanding the value of a survey, the single most important factor in establishing and maintaining a positive work environment is the first-line supervisor. This individual comes in direct, daily contact with the people providing services to the customers. The level of fairness, empathy, relationship building, common sense, enthusiasm and consistency of this individual is critically important to the organization. Workers look up to this first-line supervisor, and the value of the worker/supervisor relationship is directly proportional to the morale of the work environment. The selection and training of the first-line supervisor is critical to establishing and maintaining a positive work environment.

7. Retain the best.

Think back to the people who left your practice in the past two years. Make two lists. First, list the people who left when you wanted them to stay (the "Keep" list), and second, list those people who left and you were happy they left (the "Go" list).

Now ask yourself "Why did the Keepers leave?" Was it money, better job, moved, hours, commute, whatever? What could you have done to maintain this talent? Certainly, they were highly trained and performing up to standards. Perhaps an employee survey or honest exit interview discussions might lead to retaining top talent.

On the other side, look at the people on the "Go" list. Look at who hired them. Find out if these people were bad hires or if something happened to them in their work experience that changed their attitude toward the practice. Chances are something happened and management has to take responsibility for the work experience and environment.

No matter what your analysis reveals, the point is that attracting and maintaining talent is a key competitive edge for the organization. The better the team, the (consistently) higher the performance of the organization becomes.

The service industry, whether hotels, restaurants or resorts, is much like the health care industry. The common denominator is people—people taking care of people. Organizations with a reputation for high levels of service, such as RCHC, Darden Restaurants and Disney, have a clear focus on attracting and maintaining their customers, internal and external. It is this reputation as a great place to work and as a caring service provider that, once earned, is your best competitive edge in the marketplace.

Case Study: Ritz-Carlton

Over the past decade, health care organizations have begun to place a tremendous emphasis on viewing themselves as service providers. Journals and national symposiums have focused extensively on making patients the center of care.

Naturally, this has had an effect on how medical practices conduct business. For instance, a hospital CEO in Fort Collins, CO, works the night shift in different departments to better understand the role and problems his employees face. Some OBs and GYNs have customized their practices to focus closely on meeting the lifestyle needs of patients. In a sincere—and admirable—effort to accommodate their patients, these physicians have adjusted their office hours, set up phone triage systems, dedicated special resource and consultation rooms for female health education, and located these rooms adjacent to other important family services.

On the other hand, many consumer businesses excel at providing service. Walt Disney World prides itself on being the entertainment capital of the world. They employ many hourly workers who are the front-line contact with their guests. When a family enters Walt Disney World, its expectations are very high. Sometimes, they have saved several years to make the trek to Orlando. And most of the time, through hard work and resource management, their expectations are exceeded.

What does that mean for health care? It's means there are models out there that we can emulate as we deal with our customers and attempt to meet their needs.

In Chapter 5, you'll meet Richard Harris, whose story provides an excellent example of staff empowerment. As you'll see, it also illustrates outstanding customer service.

Harris was forced to commute extensively to Cleveland over a one-year period to receive health care for his unusual cancer. On his first visit, he decided to stay at the Ritz-Carlton located downtown. He made his reservation over the Internet, and when he compared prices, he found the Ritz-Carlton to be competitive with most of the other quality downtown hotels.

Since price was not an issue, Harris selected a familiar brand. He could have stayed at the Omni, the Sheraton or the Renaissance, as their prices were within $15 of each other. Based on his past experience and the company's image, Harris knew that the Ritz-Carlton prided itself on customer service. And because he knew that he was going to have two surgeries and be involved in a clinical trial, he wanted to develop a long-term relationship with the hotel in which he would live during those times.

Once the date was set for his first surgery, Harris placed a call to the general manager of the hotel. Explaining that he would be in the Cleveland area for his first visit for approximately two weeks, Harris indicated that he would like to stay with them during his recovery from surgery. The general manager welcomed Harris, asked what special needs he might have and assured him that the entire staff would be available to serve him as they do all guests.

Four days before his arrival in Cleveland, Harris received a phone call from the hotel. He was asked if he anticipated having any needs that might be out of the ordinary when he returned to the hotel after surgery. The guest relations person on the phone suggested the hotel would provide a room with both a shower and bathtub. She also suggested that they could provide a small stool for the bathtub to make it easier for Harris to get in and out of the tub until he was cleared to take a shower. Finally, she gave him her phone extension number and asked him to call her if there was anything that any of the Ritz-Carlton staff could do to make his stay easier.

When Harris had to return to Cleveland for his second surgery, again he called the general manager at the Ritz-Carlton. The general manager asked Harris if he liked his previous room and would like to go back there again. He also told Harris that because he was becoming such a frequent guest, he would like to offer him complimentary use of the Ritz Club. This amenity definitely added value to Harris' hotel stay, allowing him access to a quiet area with food presentations throughout the day and a host or hostess who became familiar with Harris' daily regimen.

Harris was particularly pleased that every employee at the Ritz-Carlton offered a quiet but personal greeting whenever they saw him or any other guest. That greeting was often the only time Harris heard his name spoken during his visit. Although he was extremely pleased with the care he got at the Cleveland Clinic, Harris still was away from his home, family and friends.

He was in Cleveland for what seemed like a long period of time, under less than ideal conditions, and it could have been very isolating.

Instead, every staff person at the Ritz-Carlton made a point of acknowledging Harris' existence through eye contact, a smile, a helping hand and an interest in his well-being. No matter where he went in the hotel, Harris felt as if people cared about how his day was going and if his needs were being met as he recovered. This, he felt, was about people caring for people, not about the price of a room. It represented an outstanding level of excellent employee/guest service.

For example, Harris was very grateful for the service he received from the doormen and the bellmen. They were gentle with him as he got in and out of taxicabs to go to the Clinic. Upon his return from surgery, they offered to help him walk to his room. He never felt that this was about gratuities, but more about caring for a guest who was at their hotel under unusual and complicated times.

The housekeeping staff reached out to him as professionals in their field— and as human beings. They had the opportunity to observe Harris in his room as he was fighting his battle against cancer. He was vulnerable, living in a hotel, and for his own emotional well-being, trying to live as normally as possible.

Although the staff worked hard to do a good job, one particular housekeeper exceeded Harris' expectations. She continuously looked for ways to provide him with meaningful service. For instance, she took it upon herself to provide extra pillows so he could support his body after surgery.

After his second surgery, this housekeeper knew he had been discharged from the hospital only three days post-op. In his hotel room, he had to deal with drains, dressing changes and limited mobility. Each morning, she asked what his schedule would be like the next day as well as when he would like to have his linens changed and his room tidied.

That short, seemingly insignificant conversation gave Harris a sense that he had control over his schedule, which was important as he strove to maintain a positive attitude about his cancer and his post-op recovery. That housekeeper was empowered to do what was best for the guest.

One day she said to him, " Sir, I apologize if I am out of line, but I think I know what you're going through. I lost a daughter to kidney cancer. I requested to work with your room because I want to bring positive and good things to you while you stay with us at the Ritz-Carlton."

Some people may think that as a housekeeper, she overstepped her bounds. To Harris, it conveyed a sense of extended family, rather than the isolation of being a guest and living in a hotel in a vacuum.

When Harris knew he had to return to Cleveland for over a month to participate in the clinical trial, he again called the general manager at the Ritz-Carlton. He explained the situation and received heartfelt concern. Again he was asked, "What is the best way we can help you while you're here?"

You may think that Harris was paying an exorbitant price to be a guest in the hotel and have exceptional service. Well, he did indeed experience exceptional service, but he paid a price competitive with other quality downtown hotels in the Cleveland market. For him, the issue was having service he could count on and the sense that people knew and cared about what he was going through. This was especially important as he became more focused on his disease and relationships became more important.

Each Ritz-Carlton staff person went out of his or her way to welcome Harris back to the hotel and ask if there was anything that could be done, on or off property, that would help him. Harris felt comfortable informing the general manager and some of the other key administrative people about his therapy and how ill he could become from the side effects. He didn't feel he was just a guest. Instead, he felt as if he really mattered to the hotel staff. He knew they didn't want to change places with him, but they did want to ease his suffering if they could.

In the beginning of the clinical trial, Harris had to be at the Cleveland Clinic every day. One of the doormen suggested that Harris could hire a driver for about the same fee as a cab ride. However, the car could be scheduled in advance, and it would never smell from secondhand smoke, which was particularly annoying to Harris. This arrangement worked out very well. In fact, upon hearing the circumstances, the driver offered to run errands that would make Harris' life a bit easier while he was away from home.

One day, the general manager telephoned Harris and told him that employees had asked at the staff meeting if there were other things they could do to help Harris while he was a guest. One of the bellmen related how he'd recommended a very responsible driver to ease the transportation back and forth to the Clinic. And when the general manager explained the other purpose for his call, it really surprised Harris.

The general manager was calling to make the hotel car available for Harris' use on the days he went to the Clinic for an hour visit versus a six-hour treatment. He told Harris that all he had to do was let the manager on duty know what time he would need the car, and it would be their pleasure to make it available. He told Harris that everyone in the hotel was concerned about his well-being and wished him a speedy recovery. Harris felt this was certainly the epitome of service and thoughtfulness—and it represented a level of caring that went far beyond a simple night's room rental.

Every day, Harris received a call from the in-house dining department. The spokesperson asked, "Sir, is there anything we can do to make your stay more pleasant today?"

One day, Harris was feeling very ill from the anti-cancer medicine he received in the clinical trial. It was a gloomy day, and he was feeling discouraged about everything. As he looked out the window on this gray, cold day, he replied, "Well, if you could make it 80 degrees and tropical outside, that might help." The hotel spokesperson laughed and said, "I'm not sure I can control the weather. But, if there's anything else, please call us."

About an hour later, there was a knock on the door. Harris' wife answered it only to see a room service waiter. "Oh, there must be a mistake," she said. " We didn't order anything." The server told her, "This is a treat from room service to you. We can't change the weather, but we thought these frozen pina coladas and this magazine article about the Caribbean islands would be a step in the right direction."

Both Harrises were speechless. Once again, an empowered Ritz-Carlton employee saw an opportunity and took advantage of it to provide value and service to a guest.

During the month that the Harrises were in Cleveland, they celebrated their 33rd wedding anniversary. This was difficult, as both of them silently wondered what the following year would bring, since his disease continued to be a focal point their life. Since Harris was having a fairly good day, they went outside for a walk.

Upon their return, they entered their room to see a huge, beautiful bouquet of spring flowers. They looked at the card which said, "Happy anniversary from the ladies and gentlemen of the Ritz-Carlton." It was quite a surprise, and it meant a great deal, especially since the Harrises were away from friends and family on their special day.

Later in the day, Mrs. Harris asked one of the staff how they knew it was their anniversary. She was told that a fax had come in wishing them a happy anniversary, and once the staff found out about it, they all wanted to help the Harrises celebrate.

After a while, as a result of the anti-cancer treatment, Harris lost his sense of taste and his appetite. His doctors encouraged him to feed his body small amounts every few hours, rather than think of dining in particular. But Harris just wasn't interested. His wife went down to the main dining room and met with the service staff there and asked for their help. Over and over, she received the same answer. "We'll be happy to help any way we can." Regardless of what was on the menu, the chef assured her he was willing to prepare light meals that Harris could tolerate.

Whenever Harris had a concern, two things always happened. No matter which employee he spoke to—from the bellmen to the Ritz Club management—all behaved as ladies and gentlemen. They took pride and honor in their jobs. And everyone Harris encountered exhibited behavior that indicated ownership of the problem and the responsibility for resolving it.

Prior to returning home, Harris met with the general manager one final time to explain how much he appreciated the service and care he'd received during his stay. He asked, "How do you motivate your staff? These are young people, earning an hourly wage, wearing a uniform and yet so motivated to provide excellent service."

The general manager said, "We invest in our staff because we understand that they are the most important people here. They are the ones who interact most with our guests. They deliver the service, sell our product and provide essential support in many ways.

"We work very hard to share information so that our employees can do a better job. We also hire the right staff, and we provide job security, training and good pay. It all serves to ensure that our guests will choose to return to a Ritz-Carlton hotel."

He continued, "We find that employees recognize the investment we make in them. Because they feel a sense of control over their work areas, they develop skills that help them on the job, and they accept empowerment and responsibility. Our work force has come together to serve a single goal. They understand we are in the business of assisting our guests and taking care of other human beings."

This very personal story is a phenomenal example of outstanding customer service. Do we do it this way in health care? In my experience, rarely. Instead, we hire hourly workers, put them in uniforms and think we've accomplished our goal. Sure, sometimes we "talk the talk" of patient service. But do we provide it?

Until we empower, train and build skills, we have not done our jobs. I believe we can learn a lot from the hospitality and entertainment industries—important lessons that can translate into sound service skills in the health care industry.

Chapter 2

Understanding Your Customers

"No matter what kind of business you're in, the people around you don't accept what you say at face value. They watch what you do for clues to your real priorities and concerns. If the boss dodges unpleasant duties, leaves customers on hold, communicates poorly or not at all, or otherwise shrugs off customer concerns, employees will do the same. Soon, customers will notice that the only kind of service they're getting is lip service. In no time at all, they'll be someone else's customers."

—Dick Schaaf and Ron Zemke, *Taking Care of Business*

Why worry about customer service anyway? In fact, why market at all? If you open an office, the patients will come. Right?

Obviously, that's what some physicians think. Many feel they have no control over what's going on these days. They figure: why spend good money investing in their practices when managed care is so strong? After all, how can anything they do make a difference when the insurance companies are so influential about how health care is now delivered?

These physicians have come to believe, perhaps rightly so, that today's health care is mostly about finance, rather than patient care.

Remember, just a few years ago, popular wisdom had it that managed care would take away all choice for patients. However, patients wouldn't tolerate that. Having been educated about their rights by both television and print media, they stood up to their employers and the big insurance companies. And they won. They fought for and got what they want—control, choice, quality.

Fortunately, they also want physicians who will guide them toward appropriate and safe health care. They want leaders who genuinely appreciate customers' needs and who will make them a top priority.

How do you accomplish this? Where do you start?

One way to begin is to make sure you first know who your customers are and what they want. Whether they are patients, employers, managed care administrators, referring physicians—or anyone else with whom you do business—they're all your customers. And, they all have specific needs and expectations from your practice.

Patients

When you think about marketing, you should first concentrate on meeting the needs of patients. Obviously, their needs can vary from the very complex to the very simple. Although some may require a sophisticated response, most can be easily—and inexpensively—met.

Patients/employees who are purchasing managed care benefits or are selecting a health plan want to find providers with whom they are familiar. They want their fears and concerns addressed. Having heard or read that reform will give them less choice, they're concerned that gatekeepers will reduce health care resources to save money or to line their own pockets.

They also look for familiarity, trust and name recognition. They want to believe that they're with the really good quality doctors on the managed care panels their employers select. They want to believe that quality doctors have reduced their overhead to become lean and mean through business operations, rather than by withholding clinical resources.

The following list is compiled from the results of numerous focus groups and interviews with patients prior to facilitating many group practice strategic planning sessions. Although it is not all inclusive, it will give you an good idea of patient desires. Note that many of the items are related to what is of value to the patient who uses the services and the expertise provided by medical practices:
- Patients want to be able to reach you when they need you;
- Patients want the phone answered by a person with a friendly voice who understands the nature and urgency of their problem;
- Patients want to know how long it will take for someone to return a phone call;

- Patients also want other information, such as:
- Do you accept my insurance?
- What will happen to me during my visit?
- When will I have results of diagnostic tests?
- Can I send e-mail to my doctor?
- Does the practice have a Web page?

Following are a few easy items that can be implemented by almost any practice in the United States. They are very basic to meeting the needs of those with whom you do business. Think of this as a review chart—an exercise checklist to be included in your environmental assessment:

- Be sure your reception area is a pleasant, tidy area for patients. Provide patients with a phone to make local calls;
- Provide coffee or fruit juice for patients and visitors in your reception area;
- Update magazines in your reception area so they are no more than 90 days old. Have a subscription to the daily paper available for patients to read;
- Create a display in the reception area that highlights your physicians by photo and specialty. Patients enjoy knowing what their physician looks like prior to their first meeting;
- Develop a one-page fact sheet that describes your physician providers, your subspecialties and the services available within your group;
- Have one-page articles available to provide health education. This can include seasonal information as well as facts about procedures or screenings available within your practice;
- Place long-lasting fresh flowers in your reception area at the beginning of each week. At the end of the week, invite patients to take flowers as they leave the practice;
- Have a suggestion box in your reception area with three-by-five cards on which patients can jot down ideas and comments to improve your practice's patient service;
- At least once a month, sit in your reception area. Use this time to read the magazines available for patients, look at the decor and notice what it's like to be a patient in your practice. Change those things that don't make you feel good about being there;
- Invest in some coloring books, paper dolls and other child-safe toys to keep children and parents happy while they're awaiting their turn to be seen;
- Make it a goal to have no patient wait longer than 15 minutes for an appointment. Encourage patients to notify your staff if the wait is longer; and
- Keep in mind the patient education tips shown in Figure 2-a.

Figure 2-a

Patient education tips

- Patients given oral instruction alone could recall 70 percent of the information three hours later. Three days later, they could recall only 10 percent.
- Patients given a visual handout could recall 72 percent of the information three hours later. Three days later, they could recall only 20 percent.
- When a blend of telling and showing was used to educate patients, they could recall 85 percent after three hours, and three days later, they could recall 65 percent of the information.
- We know patients hear, but do they listen?
- Patient education fact sheets and other educational materials help patient compliance.
- If patient compliance is improved, outcomes can be enhanced.
- When outcomes are enhanced, patient satisfaction is increased.

Employers

Employers are your customers too. They pay the bills, of course, but even more important, their employees are your patients. And, believe it or not, employers aren't monsters. It's certainly in your best interest to know them and to collaborate with them.

Employers want a hassle-free system that will satisfy their employees. Obviously, they want the best possible care, plus a lack of employee complaints. And, of course, service counts, especially in a capitated system.

Preferring not to deal with a lot of individual providers in groups, they also want:
- Accountability for services and physician selection on a panel;
- Education about what they're buying;
- Reasonable controls on pricing;
- Protection from abusive practices or billing patterns;
- Patient guidance and education; and
- Visionary development of new programs.

It's important to build relationships with employers, help them understand the role your practice plays in health care leadership and delivery in your community, as well as the leadership role you play with their employees. Building these relationships is your job. There is no one else who will do it for you.

Why not call a major employer in your community and introduce yourself as an administrator or a physician who sees a lot of their employees? Suggest going to lunch or set up a meeting for a face-to-face visit. During the meeting, your opportunity—your strategy, if you will—should be to find out about the employer's specific health care needs and how you can help the company meet those needs. Share what your practice is doing to enhance care. Let them know how your practice interacts with their employees. And answer their questions or concerns about the relationship between their employees and your practice.

If you're reluctant to do this, perhaps you should ask yourself how you can do business with people you don't talk to. If you know that there's an employer with whom you want to do business—because of size or role in the community—simply find a way to initiate a relationship. And, as you'll see as you read further, it really is not all that difficult.

Fostering a positive customer-service attitude

As you've already seen by the example in Chapter 1, customer service is an important element that will help you retain customers/patients. It's how your staff and physicians treat patients—their customer-service attitude. Studies show that when patients change doctors, it usually has nothing to do with the quality of medical care provided—except if insurers have changed.

More often than not, patients change because of how they perceive they're treated within a practice. It often has to do with something as simple as a phone or front-desk contact. That's why you can't afford to have anyone on your staff who isn't trained, motivated and empowered to meet patient demands. And it's important to remember that the attitude toward patient service frequently stems from the physicians or management of the practice.

The lesson to be learned: You can be the best physician in the world, and you can have the finest colleagues available in your group, but if you're not paying attention to customer service issues and concerns, you will lose patients.

Another lesson: doing it right the first time is far less expensive than getting patients back once they've left your practice.

How do you do it right? It can be as easy as investing in service training so that your staff can meet the needs of patients. Usually, you can find courses and in-service training right in your community. Frequently, your hospital provides them. Also, many Chambers of Commerce hold professional development training courses. Or, there are seminar leaders who focus on this type of training as they travel throughout the country.

In addition, MGMA offers courses for medical office staff. Look for those that provide customer service training for receptionists and other office workers, including subjects such as assertiveness training, how to deal with angry patients and how to communicate properly with patients.

Finally, you must strive to meet the needs of your other primary customers— managed care and referrers. Just as they were in 1994 when I wrote *Position for Success! Strategic Marketing for Group Practice,* managed care plans are usually most concerned about:
- Cost-effectiveness;
- Access;
- Quality of care;
- Privileges at participating hospitals;
- Similar philosophy;
- Customer service and satisfaction; and
- Differentiation of their provider panel.

Referring physicians, on the other hand, want their patients to receive high-quality care and to have their patients referred back to them for follow-up care. In addition, they want prompt, informative reports and appropriate, cost-effective tests. They also want to work with specialists who will adapt to efficient and cost-effective care management. Further information about working with referrers is provided in Chapter 7.

Before you can hope to develop an efficient, effective marketing program, it's vital that you completely understand yourself and your practice. To do this, you must carefully assess your practice—both internally and externally—with the goal being to develop a clear understanding of your market, as well as learn how to negotiate and monitor managed care contracts.

Ask yourself how you're doing. Are you meeting those needs? Have you empowered your staff? Have you tooled your organization so that patients and other customers see you as a customer service provider, not just a quality health care provider?

The following chapters will help you answer these and other important questions regarding how to market your group practice.

Figure 2-b

Sample service statement

Our medical practice will do everything possible to help provide our patients with superior services, innovative thinking and efficient operations. We know that our success and our survival depend on how well we consistently serve our customers whenever they are involved with our practice. We understand that each employee's job has an impact on the timeliness, quality, empathy and service that we offer. We will respect and have concern for our patients' needs. We understand that one negative patient encounter is one error too many. We will strive to do our job right the first time and to continually seek performance improvement.

Case study: Radiology

I worked with one major community employer who was very concerned about what his self-insured company was spending on MRI. For the first time in the history of the company, they were spending more on MRI than obstetrics.

One radiology group practice stood out as being the largest provider of imaging care for that employer. Not surprisingly, the employer began to wonder if this imaging group was in some way over-utilizing MRI because their name was on a high percentage of his bills. He was not educated that radiologists do not order exams but instead, only interpret them.

I asked this employer if he understood how MRI was involved in diagnosis. I also asked if he had a relationship with a radiology group. He was very knowledgeable about his company's health care expenditures and about which groups of physicians were providing care to his employees. He was so frustrated with the high expense of MRI that he believed something was amiss and wanted to put MRI services out for bid in the community.

Instead, I suggested that perhaps the first step would be to meet with the radiology group and ask for education about the technology and use of MRI. The employer was willing to do that. Simultaneously, the managing doctor of the imaging group was delighted to have a chance to meet with an employee benefits manager. The employee benefits manager asked permission to bring two of his industrial nurses on the visit.

The date and time was set, a map was sent, and the radiologist suggested the employer set aside two hours for the visit. When the employer and his nurses began their tour and visit at the MRI center, the clinical radiologist on duty was reading a MRI of the brain that had been ordered for a patient with severe headaches. He was able to discuss the case he was viewing with the guests. He explained that the patient had a tumor in a very unusual place. They held discussions about how many tests and how many physicians that patient had seen before having the MRI as the ultimate diagnostic tool.

They also discussed how much time the employee/patient had probably missed from his job due to illness and doctor appointments. They were able to have a discussion about the cost-effectiveness of MRI over other traditional x-ray and diagnostic examinations. And a dialog took place that allowed the employer to have a much greater appreciation of the uses of MRI in diagnosis.

When the employer expressed his frustration at his high bills for MRI, a discussion occurred about who orders diagnostic exams and what role the radiologist plays in educating referring physicians about appropriateness of utilizing these tools. The radiologist communicated that there is no good mechanism for teaching referring physicians about the appropriateness of ordering exams. But he also was able to tell the employer that in their community, the radiology specialists were working with the insurers and primary care physicians to try to change behaviors based on the new technology available in imaging. And so these two people, the employer who pays the bills and the radiologist who interprets the exams began developing a relationship.

The marketing involved included the radiology group sharing with the employer information, education and a tour of the MRI center. This tour, in turn, lent itself to an enhanced opportunity. The managing partner was comfortable suggesting that the employer and the nurses also tour some of the other areas of imaging that their employees used on a daily basis for disease diagnosis or treatment.

The next stop was the mammography department. The employer learned that this radiology group was very focused on quality assurance. And because of that focus, the group had put in a system of double reads for mammography. The managing partner providing the tour was honest and upfront in explaining the dilemma of mammography. He was able to explain that mammography has become a wonderful screening tool for breast cancer. But it is not an exact science, and errors are sometimes made because of the difficulty in reading mammography at 100 percent accuracy.

He shared with the employer that their radiology group was subspecialized and those who read mammography do it as an area of specialization. He shared the huge volume that goes through their department. He also educated the employer about the kinds of mammography equipment in which the group had invested. He told the employer all that the group had done to create a very fine mammography department. He emphasized that they still do double reads to try to eliminate errors in diagnosis and evaluation.

The employer asked who pays for the double reads. The radiologist said, "You don't." He explained, "This is our approach to practicing good medicine. This is our choice about how to run our practice for the women in our community."

Following the mammography department tour, the managing partner walked the employer and the nurses over to the pediatric and women's hospital. He took them to the area of the Fetal Diagnostic Center where he explained that it's a lot less expensive and a lot less traumatic to patients if they understand their options when they have a high likelihood of delivering a baby with problems.

The radiologist explained that the technology in ultrasound is very sophisticated. When a patient has an ultrasound and it looks like there is a problem in the pregnancy, she is referred to the Fetal Diagnostic Center. The pregnancy is tracked to understand what problems the baby will likely have at birth. The parents meet with a perinatologist, the genetic counselor and the radiologist. Counseling is done to help plan for the birth of the baby.

During the remainder of the pregnancy, the patient revisits the Fetal Diagnostic Center to track the baby's development. The plus side and cost-effective side of this is that when that baby is birthed, there will be a plan of action to give that baby its greatest chance at life in the most effective way. Sometimes that means going to the operating room immediately after delivery. Because the baby's physical needs are planned for, the family enjoys the greatest opportunity for a good outcome.

After the Fetal Diagnostic Center, the tour continued on to the Angio Interventional Lab. It was explained that angio interventional radiology has become an area of diagnosis, treatment and intervention into disease. They observed a patient having a procedure. They watched the radiologist communicate with the patient and observed the procedure on television monitors while outside the lab.

The radiologist brought the employer to this area to show that, when it's appropriate, there are cost-effective and new approaches for treating patients, rather than surgery. The radiologist explained the relationship between referring physicians such as vascular surgeons, general surgeons and oncologists, in determining the most appropriate referral during a patient's disease.

At the end of a couple of hours, the group sat together having refreshments. They agreed that it had been an important day for the doctors, the employers and their patients. The employer had a whole new appreciation of what happens to their employees when they're referred to this radiology group inside this hospital system. And a business relationship that had simply been an exchange of paper, which evolved into resentment over dollars spent, was changed by the interface between the physician who is the diagnostician and caregiver and the employer who is funding the process.

In fact, a relationship was built so quickly that the employer asked the radiologist if he could spend some time reviewing the appropriateness of the MRI referrals of his employees.   The employer wanted to know what percentage of referrals was appropriate and how often referring physicians were not utilizing imaging appropriately. The radiologist said, "Sure, we'd be happy to help." That step has not yet taken place, but the request for help and the positive response helped build an even more solid relationship.

What happened in this example? Two people who had been doing business together but had never met, learned much about each other. They expressed consideration for each other's needs and explained how those needs were being met. This relationship between physician group and employer matured and was personalized at a very rapid rate.

The employer now has a new awareness of how his dollars are being spent. He also had an awareness of the role the radiologist plays in the case management of his employees' care. The foundation of a new relationship was built. And some of the concerns about the radiologists being frivolous with the employer's health care dollars were dispelled.

There has never been another question from this major employer about the imaging bills. However, there has been an ongoing relationship between that employer and the managing partner of the radiology group. The benefits person now feels comfortable calling the radiologist to ask for help in understanding appropriateness of care for some employees who have been critically injured or ill.

This example is all about understanding your customers—developing relations with people with whom you do business. It's called relationship marketing.

Figure 2-c

How to Build Better Customer Service

1. Make customer service a priority, but first make sure that everyone you employ knows what service means and how it should be carried out within your practice.

2. Give customers extra value. Find ways to recognize long-time patients and referrers for their loyalty to your practice. This can be as simple as a personal handwritten note from the physician.

3. No matter what the size of your group, information systems and documentation are critical. By keeping records of patients and referring physicians, you can identify trends that foretell customers' changing needs. And, don't just read reports. Take action from the information you extract from them. Assign someone to review trend reports and recommend actions for the group.

4. Use technology, because it's as important as intellectual capital in today's complex world.

5. Pay attention to all components of your practice, not to just the external side the patients see. Your infrastructure, processes, systems and people support the culture of your organization.

6. Don't compromise on quality in products, services and people. Especially people.

7. Find out what your customers experience at your practice. Hire a mystery shopper to become your mystery patient and have that person evaluate interactions and experiences, then report back to your group.

8. Track and identify the department that reports the most patient complaints each month. Use the staffing in that area of your practice to help come up with solutions.

9. Reward staff who communicate problems and patient concerns. You want them to reveal any mistakes they make, rather than hide them for fear of disciplinary action.

10. No matter how briefly your staff interacts with patients or other customers, train them to use the patient's or customer's name. Your goal is to have everyone who interacts with your practice treated as if they are important to your practice.

11. Every chance you get, demonstrate your commitment to customer service, thoroughly and intently, to your staff, your patients and others with whom you do business. Seek anecdotes, opinions and surveys from your patients, vendors, and competitors that will allow you to enhance your service.

12. Experience your competitors. Find out what they offer that could attract managed care or employers to do business with them rather than with your practice.

Figure 2-d

Cleveland Clinic service statement

The Cleveland Clinic Foundation has worked very hard to provide service to all patients in all departments. As a guest in their facility, I noticed the following document posted in a nursing station, and I asked for a copy to share with you. The Clinic has found a way to empower its staff, both by training and by the following reminder.

Excel in Service

Show respect and courtesy in every encounter:
- Stop what you are doing and extend a warm welcome;
- Greet everyone with a smile, make eye contact, use their name whenever possible and ask how you may assist them;
- Listen intensively and ask questions to confirm your understanding;
- Respond to requests and take responsibility for addressing the needs of others; and
- Practice courteous telephone etiquette.

Show empathy when you are communicating:
- Acknowledge the person, situation and feelings;
- Avoid excuses; deliver what you promise;
- Keep everyone well informed; clearly communicate the plan of care/action;
- Offer options; invite involvement in resolving requests; and
- Guide the patients through our system to the appropriate resources.

Show cooperation, professionalism and pride in your job:
- Be honest; promise only what you can deliver;
- Respond quickly to requests and insure tasks are completed accurately and on time;
- Respect the confidentiality of all patients and colleagues;
- Talk positively about other employees and departments within the presence of patients and visitors; and
- Create a positive environment in your appearance, attitude and behavior.

Chapter **3**

Back to Basics

*"We all grow up one day. A **business plan** tells others what we will be when we grow up. A **strategic plan** sets the path that we will take. A **marketing plan** outlines how glorious our trip will be."*

—Ed Cabrera, MD, MBA

At this point, you may be asking: Exactly what is medical marketing anyway? How is it done? What benefits does it have for me?

Marketing a medical practice is, for the most part, just like marketing any other business. Naturally, we have our own set of circumstances, but when it comes right down to it, most of the textbook tenets of marketing still apply. If you're at all uncertain about how to go about it, I've included a number of excellent resources at the end of this book.

That said, I think it's important to review a few basics before we proceed. Let's start by looking at the differences between a business plan, a strategic plan and a marketing plan.

A **business plan** lays out your company's direction, vision and mission. It's important because it defines your organization, your goals and your objectives. It details your current financial position and projects what you expect it to be in the future (usually five years down the road).

Your business plan serves as an objective course for your organization. Internally, it provides direction for the leadership, and externally it is a vital step in your pursuit of debt or equity financing.

In essence, a business plan describes your business in intimate detail. It is very important that you take it seriously if you want to achieve your stated goals.

A *strategic plan* takes a long, hard look at your goals and objectives. It outlines your strengths and weakness as well as your opportunities and the possible threats to your practice. It details a plan of action with expected results, along with contingencies for the unexpected. It permits your organization to plan effectively the pursuit of your goals in an objective fashion. A strategic plan complements your business plan and is augmented by your marketing plan.

Finally, your *marketing plan* serves as the blueprint for the marketing actions of your group. Encompassing advertising, promotion, image and mind-set, it can determine how efficient and effective you will be in generating revenues, and it definitely impacts sales. In fact, it can mark the difference between just "getting by" and being very successful.

Why market?

Obviously change and consolidation over the past decade have impacted all of health care. We've all watched our environment move from hospitals and management companies acquiring practices to those same entities disengaging from their acquisitions.

However, a few areas have remained constant. It's still important to come together as a group, define your specific practice goals and make a group commitment to move toward those goals. It's still important to differentiate yourself from the rest of the pack and build your own brand name identity.

So what does marketing accomplish? It allows you to know who your customers are, understand what they want and give them the products and services that your group has to offer.

Why market? It provides the road map that allows you to:
- Develop brand name identity;
- Differentiate from colleagues;
- Shore up internal relations;
- Enhance patient service;
- Develop partner relations with employers;
- Enhance relations with managed care;
- Develop relationships with the media; and
- Commit to service for all customers at all times.

Of course, the ideal situation is to hold a retreat, develop strategic goals and then develop a marketing plan to achieve those goals. Obviously, not all groups do that.

Some practices use a consultant to develop a marketing plan, without the benefit of a strategic planning retreat. Others find their own ways to develop specific marketing goals and choose to implement a plan of action or campaign without the benefit of a retreat or a comprehensive marketing plan.

In any case, it is important to understand the benefits of a written marketing plan or at the very least, a written plan of action. The operative word here is written. It is very important to commit your plan to paper so you have a clearly defined, written document to reflect upon as you work to achieve your goals.

Let's face it. We're all in the same boat these days. The marketplace has changed because of the consolidation that continues to impact health care. But we must remember that health care is practiced on a local level. In some communities, the situation is more difficult than others. But the basics still apply. We should do what we do because we've designed and planned it—because it's the right thing for our group in our community.

Working with managed care

First, let's agree on this: in today's health care world, working with managed care companies must be considered a basic element of marketing. They have become a customer in line with referring physicians and patients. They represent the initial hurdle that has to be cleared in a managed care setting. Obviously, being excluded from the network excludes your group from seeing patients represented by the managed care plan.

In addition, managed care companies are not the enemy. In any case, you must learn to deal with them—because they're here to stay as we enter the new millennium.

However, all organizations do not deal with managed care in the same manner. Typically, those having smaller panels of participating physicians require primary care physicians to be gatekeepers and to authorize referrals. Most require pre-certification for hospitalization, approval for some specialty care by a medical director, and many include fee withholds with a variety of risk arrangements. All have ongoing review in quality assurance activities.

Building relationships is the most important key to positioning today's medical practices for successful managed care. Toward that goal, it's important to note there are areas within a managed care organization that are very important to maintaining

ongoing, productive relationships with a group practice. They are:
- Utilization management;
- Provider relations;
- Member services/satisfaction; and
- Ability to be price friendly.

The lesson learned from saturated managed care markets: It's imperative that practices develop relationships with managed care. Once managed care plans have good relationships with providers, they try to maintain them.

What do managed care plans want from their relationships?
- Responsiveness;
- Price;
- Patient satisfaction;
- Quality improvement process;
- Clinical guidelines; and
- Published outcomes.

Other important factors include:
- Cost-effective behavior;
- Geographic coverage;
- Privileges at participating hospitals;
- Philosophical accord;
- Willingness to work collaboratively to develop organized systems of care with other appropriate physicians;
- Understanding of how managed care plans do business and why they do it that way;
- Practices which are willing to develop long-term partnerships; and
- Practices which can differentiate their value.

It's also very important to develop and maintain productive working relationships with two key influencers within the managed care organization: the health plan administrator and the medical director. Over time, you'll also develop relations with people within the managed care plan on multiple levels. These include sales and marketing coordinators, those in contracting and finance and those in claims.

These are the people who make decisions regarding:
- Expansion of the plan and its panel;
- Practices with whom they will contract;
- Practices which they will terminate; and
- Practices with whom they will negotiate.

What does this mean to your practice?

Once you enter into a managed care contract, you can't just stop there. You must keep working to develop the relationship further. It's important to interact frequently with medical directors. As an example, you should position proactively to assist them with their needs. Find out how you can help them reach their goals. As you may realize, this is the exact opposite of the traditional physician attitude of "This is what we do, and we are great at it. You should be grateful to work with us."

It's productive to share your cost-reduction strategies with your managed care partners, both current and future. Volunteer to participate on and even lead meetings with your managed care partners and fellow referring physicians on Organized Systems of Care. Organized Systems of Care is a collaborative approach of typically connected primary care physicians and specialists who develop disease management programs. Result: The appropriate outcome for reducing waste and duplication between physicians in various ancillary services and improved outcomes in patient health status.

Coalitions

One of the most important trends in health care today's environment is the rapid growth of business coalitions around a country. As an example, the national business coalition on health in Washington, DC, has over 100 members representing almost 35 states and 8,000 employers who, in turn, cover 35 million employees and their dependents.

Coalitions seek value, which boils down to quality plus cost-effectiveness—things that are easy to state, yet often difficult to measure. Coalitions are committed to shared values, which involve both community-based reform and value-based purchasing. Of course, there are diverse approaches, and each is at a different stage of maturity at this time. However, it's safe to state that they come together in a community for one or more of the following reasons:
- To contract for health services;
- To develop and share information;
- To improve the quality of health care services in their community;
- To educate consumers;
- To improve the health of the community; and
- To lead the business community in rallying to address health care issues.

Community-based reform means that health care is delivered locally, and purchasers and consumers demand accountability. Also, a local presence enriches local relationships and the individual commitments to them.

In value-based purchasing, consumers and purchasers will seek to maximize their value, given information on the price and quality of health care services. You should investigate what role you can and should play with your local coalition. Research the value of joining as a provider group and explore the culture of communicating about "value added" and the benefits of your community-based practice to the coalition.

Design a relationship so that you can maximize on meeting the wants and needs of the coalition as it explores the costs to employees and dependents. My experience with these groups indicates that you should gain their recognition, offer to collaborate and assist them on projects. As you develop interactive relationships, your group practice benefits by the relationship. The newly formed interaction gains the practice an important connection to benefits managers, human relations people, managed care and employee referrals.

It is very important for providers to position themselves to get on the "same sheet of music" with employers and managed care plans. In doing so, physicians can participate in addressing health care expenditures as common problems and initiate mutually rewarding solutions, to the benefit of all involved. This is especially true with chronic, debilitating diseases. Providers can add value to payers by finding ways to reduce payer costs without reducing payer prices. Payers will listen to the vision that high-quality care is ultimately less expensive. Quality providers have fewer complications and offer disease management as an approach to promote health and fewer health expenses.

In the most basic way, the partnership between you and managed care should:
- Build alliances;
- Provide an easy way to work together;
- Respond honestly and openly with each other;
- Follow the rules;
- Submit applications on time; and
- Accept changes gracefully.

The goal for employers and their employees as well as physicians is to provide services for care under contract and to develop a comprehensive network of physicians to provide that care. When utilization of care is managed effectively, money can be saved. Employers have come to understand that managed care companies often can provide necessary care to their employees in a less costly and more efficient and effective manner. And that's what they expect from both the managed care company and the physicians providing care.

There is much to be said for your ability to read managed care contracts and decide if the contract is acceptable to your group. As many of you have learned after years of contracting with managed care, you don't have to accept every contract. You don't have to remain an active member in all managed care plans with which you have contracted. There will be times when your contract is so unacceptable to the group that you choose to withdraw from that provider panel. These issues are operational in nature and usually have to do with reimbursement.

Let's assume that you are involved in a relationship with a managed care provider. What marketing opportunities are available to build value into your relationship with the managed care provider?

It's important that you provide data to demonstrate how you deliver high quality care. It's important to share the cost-effective services that your practice has developed on many administrative levels within the managed care organization. This includes the medical director, provider relation's representative, administrator, quality assurance nurse and sales reps, to name a few.

In defining your value, it's important to emphasize the board certification and fellowship training of the physicians within your organization. More than just a credentialing process, this is another way to position your group. In defining your value, also look at other opportunities to discuss ways you've enhanced the operations of the group to offer other services to referring physicians and patients.

As you develop relations with new managed care providers in town, do just that: develop a relationship. You may or may not have a contractual relationship with them. With the speed with which consolidations are taking place, it is in your best interest to know what managed care plans are offering and who their key people are in your community.

Welcome them to your office. Collaborate with them to achieve what's best for the community. Recognize that there are differences between managed care and a physician's practice. You're not in a real "marriage" at that point, but rather are working on a relationship. Make a decision that your practice will work collaboratively whenever possible.

Suppose you're in a very competitive specialty, such as cardiology, orthopaedics or oncology and recognize that the panel is going to be limited. Take time when meeting with the medical director or provider representative to be sure they know what differentiates your practice from others. Understand that this will ultimately be a contractual relationship based on finance, risk, capitation and other issues. But, you still can work to position your practice to your advantage.

Exactly what differentiates your practice from others in your market area? Begin with the marketing tasks you have developed to improve compliance from your patients. Although not limited to these, you certainly might include any or all of the following if they apply:

- Our practice conducts patient surveys and shares the results with individual physicians who have been identified for both good or negative behavior, as well as our physicians as a group. We also share survey reports with our staff. We run our survey one month a quarter.

- We establish a patient compliance record which is reviewed by our administrator and our managing physician. We use patient complaints for counseling purposes to coach our staff and enhance patient relations. We ask our staff how they would solve the problem if they were the patients.

- When we expand our practice to additional office sites, we do a marketing plan of action to communicate with both existing patients and new patients in the expanded area. We do this as a service to both. We know there's an advantage to being close to patients when they need us.

- We review our office hours and use information received on customer surveys to determine when to establish nontraditional office hours.

- We have an ongoing committee which makes recommendations when it's time to redecorate and refresh our physical plant.

- We review our telephone policies on an annual basis. We do in-house training for our telephone staff to help them help our patients in a friendly and engaging manner. We work closely with a telecommunications consultant to have appropriate and useful telephone equipment.

- We review our office appointment policies and encourage our scheduling staff to work with our nursing staff and come up with recommendations to enhance this process.

- We do cost accounting to know what it costs us to do business.

- We have been very aggressive in finding software that helps us track services, referrals and reimbursement.

- We have a mission statement that is reviewed each year at our annual strategic planning retreat. When it's appropriate, our mission statement is defined. When the mission statement is changed, we do an in-service with our staff to be sure they all understand the goals of our practice and how those goals relate with our mission.

- We are very proactive when it comes to patient education. We create fact sheet shells, which we imprint with patient education. These fact sheet shells are used throughout the practice.

- We interact with our patients through e-mail and have a practice Website.

- We use practice extenders to provide enhanced patient care and education.

Practice identity

Prior to implementing your marketing plan, it's also important to make sure you're prepared. First, be sure you can easily differentiate your practice from your competitors and colleagues in the eyes of your community. Next, review your most fundamental communication tools. Ask yourself:

- Do we have a memorable practice name?

- Do we have a graphic identity (logo) that represents what our practice stands for?

Believe me, these two elements are as basic as it gets when it comes to projecting your desired corporate image. And they couldn't be more important to establishing a successful practice identity.

In the current age of communication, it is best to work with a graphic artist to create your practice identity. Be sure to explain the image you'd like to have for your group practice, who your patients are and how they are referred to your group. Keep in mind that the logo you are creating is for the ease of your patents and others who do business with your practice.

Unless you have an artist you're already comfortable with, it's in your best interest to ask for quotes for creating the logo and the corporate identity package from a few artists in your marketplace. In addition to price considerations, try to work with someone who is comfortable designing logos and stationery packages. Find one who is interested in working with a small business and is sensitive to your needs. And remember to ask for a timeline so you know when to expect the layout of your logo and its application on your stationery pieces.

When you ask for quotes for your stationery package, plan for the following basic items:
- Logo design;
- Logo art on floppy disk;
- Logo slick sheet;
- Letterhead;
- #10 envelope;
- Business cards for at least three names. If you need additional personalized cards, it will probably entail additional expense;
- Note card;
- Note card envelope;
- Self-stick mailing label;
- Appointment card;
- Rolodex card; and
- Fax cover sheet.

Additional communication tools you will need from your artist in the future may include:
- Patient handbook;
- Fact sheet shell design;
- Corporate brochure; and
- Practice folders.

It is very important to create a visual image that allows your patients and other clients to recognize your practice immediately. You want to stand out and differentiate from all of the others who provide care in your specialty and community.

This process begins with the creation of a logo that captures the essence of your practice. But I encourage you to keep in mind that the logo and identity are more for your customers than it is for yourself. They are the ones you want to influence.

When considering your logo, keep in mind that it is often your first opportunity to communicate an image for your organization and to create a predisposition in your favor. As you work with an artist or a graphic designer, communicate clearly what you wish to convey. Articulate what words best describe your organization. These are likely to include:
- Quality;
- Integrity;
- Attention to detail;
- Professionalism;

- Caring;
- A practice which is:
  - Up to date;
  - Efficient;
  - Experienced;
  - Knowledgeable;
  - Conscientious;
  - Innovative;
  - Friendly, caring;
  - Thorough; and
  - Reliable.

Remember these characteristics as well as the following guidelines as you work with a designer to develop a logo that truly represents your practice. Your logo should:

- Differentiate your practice from competitors through a distinct identity which contains a minimum of elements;
- Be clear and readable in all sizes from signage to one to five inches (or smaller, if needs dictate);
- Be strong enough to stand alone, as required for signage, yet simple enough to have a distinctive presence when other information should stand out (as in print advertising);
- Copy and fax well;
- Reproduce well in color, as well as black and white, for both high quality and budget printing projects; and
- Utilize no more than two timeless print styles, based on classic principles of weight, balance and proportion.

Initially, you should expect two to four logo designs presented in context—as you will probably use them—such as on your letterhead, envelope and business card. This facilitates evaluation and comparison by allowing you to visualize how the logo will work when combined with other information. In addition, it may reveal potential usage problems at an early stage.

Whenever possible, ask for your final logo art in both horizontal and vertical versions. This will give you greater flexibility as you use it for multiple purposes.

Figure 3-a

Value differentiation

Sometimes physicians and managers tell me that they really have a difficult time creating a differentiation list (the "value added" elements that set their practice apart from others). Because they do the same things everyday, they often don't see their practice as being special or unique to the clients and patients they serve. But, look around every time you go shopping. You'll see how easy it is to itemize special attributes.

Let's look at this example.

Recently, I was shopping for new two-line phones. I was impressed with the AT&T Lucent Technology Speakerphone 932. Many phones on the store shelf had the same capabilities, but those capabilities were not communicated as effectively. Let me just show you how AT&T differentiated its product by listing its values on the side of the box.

- 2-line speakerphone;
- Hands-free speakerphone;
- LCD display;
- 32 # memory;
- Auto re-dial;
- 3-party conferencing;
- Line status indicator;
- Receiver and speaker volume control;
- Hold button;
- Mute button;
- Distinctive ringing features;
- Hearing-aid compatible;;
- Flash features;
- Program pause;
- Selectable dialing; and
- Table or wall mount.

We know phones today are going to have many of these features. But in this instance, AT&T made sure that I understood what differentiated its product so I would be more likely to do business with this company.

When patients come to your office, it's very important that you fully educate them about your products and services in the same manner. If you survey your patients, you'll probably be amazed to find out how little they are aware of all the products and services provided within your practice. It's especially true in certain specialties such as orthopaedics where patients often say they went to a podiatrist because they didn't know an orthopaedic group provided foot and ankle care. Or patients who went to a chiropractor because they didn't know their sports medicine doctor's group also took care of backs.

Take time to review your practice and think about all you offer. Write it down. Not only will it help focus your marketing, it will be of value during your negotiations with other physicians, hospitals and managed care.

Case study: The surgeon opens a new office

Several years ago, I received a call from a physician who was considered mature in his market. He had been in practice in the community for 16 years, had been on the Board of the Medical Society and currently held positions at the local college and at a downtown corporate club.

This surgeon had privileges at all three hospital systems in town, but had tailored his practice to those hospitals that had specialty equipment and teams to care for his patients post-operatively. Because of the nature of his practice, all patients were physician referred. He made a decision to leave the group he was in and open his own practice as a solo. This was not an easy decision as he had been with the practice from its inception. In fact, he had acted as managing partner for five years.

The group had done an excellent job of negotiating contracts with the high volume managed care plans in the community. In addition, they had effectively marketed their practice and positioned themselves as leaders in their specialty.

The surgeon decided to allow four weeks from the time his decision was made until he was in his new office. This meant he had to find a medical office location, hire an office manager, create a marketing communication plan and re-establish himself with managed care plans in that time frame. He immediately hired three consultants on a project basis.

First, the surgeon consulted an attorney to be sure he was in compliance with his separation agreement, new lease and other issues relating to his opening a solo practice. The second person he hired was a consultant who helped him find and interview an office manager, negotiate with the managed care plans and create a checklist that was used to organize details relating to being ready for business in as short a time as possible. Once the office manager was in place, the consultant's job was diminished and within weeks fulfilled, as planned. The third consultant was a marketing manager on a 90-day basis.

They agreed that the physician had two immediate and short-term challenges. The first goal involved the need to develop a systematic approach to being in touch with past, present and soon-to-be future referring physicians. The goal was to dispel any rumors concerning why the surgeon resigned from the group and opened his own practice, and simultaneously, to encourage referrers to send patients to the new practice as it was open and immediately ready to see patients.

The second goal was to create an identity package for the new practice. As phase one, this involved creating a practice name, developing a corporate/practice identity and creating a patient handbook.

A name was selected and a graphic artist was retained to develop the logo and stationery package. While that was underway, a referral letter was created. While awaiting the printing of the letterhead, work began on the mailing list for the referral letter. It was decided to send the letter to all potential referring physicians in a five-county area. In this surgeon's case, the broad reach was important due to his specialty and his long-standing referral relations with physicians in several counties. It also was important that he begin properly positioning his new solo practice.

It was important to have the new practice identity in place as quickly as possible so the surgeon could communicate effectively and get the best outcome from the beginning. He identified his target markets as:
- Neurologists;
- Internal Medicine Specialists;
- Primary Care Physicians;
- Radiologists;
- Emergency Room Physicians;
- Orthopaedic Surgeons;

- Endocrinologists;
- Pulmonary Medicine Specialists;
- Oncology/Hematology Specialists;
- Radiation Therapists;
- Obstetricians/Gynecologists;and
- Chiropractors.

His goal was to communicate his professional change by personal letter, along with a Rolodex card and business card. Because he was trying to communicate with physicians in a five-county area, it was decided to use a mail house rather than try to have his limited staff handle the project.

The mail house was instructed to research all physicians in these specialties in the five-county area and then to purge the list to eliminate duplications. At the beginning of this campaign to introduce his new practice and image, the surgeon wanted to personalize each letter. However, he soon found it was beyond his budget to do so. Eventually, it was determined that the same outcome could be achieved if the letter was addressed to "Dear Colleague," rather than Dear Dr. Smith. The important part was the content of the letter, the letterhead with the new practice name and graphic design, and the sincere message from the surgeon.

The content of the letter: The letter began with a brief history of the surgeon's involvement in the local community. He emphasized his 15 years of practice and his appreciation for working with colleagues, interesting patients and the state-of-the-art technology provided by the local hospitals. He followed that paragraph with an emphasis on the changes in the evolution of his specialty and that he, too, was making a change that involved separating from his group and opening his own practice.

This gave him an opportunity to discuss how he had maintained his privileges at all major health systems within the community as well as his managed care contracts. He concluded the letter by asserting that he had a sincere interest in assisting his colleagues in caring for their patients. He communicated that he appreciated consultations and referrals and looked forward to developing and maintaining relationships.

Once the letter was created and approved, he looked for other ways to conduct the campaign right the first time, yet make it cost effective.

Here are the recommendations the surgeon was offered:

- Get a quote from the printer to imprint the letter on the new practice letterhead. Inquire if the printer has a high-resolution copier to achieve this while appearing as if the letter was typed or printed;

- Provide the printer with the doctor's signature on laser paper so it can be scanned onto the letter as if it were personally signed;

- Be sure to order enough letterhead to absorb this communication project and still have an adequate amount for the practice to use under usual circumstances;

- Get quotes from one or more mail houses with the following parameters:
  - Purchase list for one-time use to specified physicians in five-county area;
  - Database to be class certified and purged for duplicates;
  - Letter to be imprinted upon delivery. However, the letter will need to be folded and stuffed with a Rolodex card and business card;
  - Inkjet addresses onto envelopes; and
  - Bulk metered, sorted and delivered to the post office.

Note: The letter provided an opportunity to disseminate the Rolodex card and new business cards all at one mailing.

- Proposed budget to mail the letter and inserts:
  - List purchase of 1300 names approximately: $500;
  - Mailing services approximately: $335;
  - Postage: $329;
  - Total cost for mailing: $1164.

In sum, this project cost the surgeon $0.90 per referring physician.

This story produced a successful outcome in multiple ways. The surgeon was able to conduct damage control plus public relations branding and positioning. The personal letter, which allowed the surgeon to tell his own story, helped to control any possible gossip and to position him as he desired. By using the letter as a vehicle for his Rolodex and business cards, he ensured no breakdown in communication for referring physicians.

> Within days of his letter being delivered, he was delighted to receive personal notes and flower arrangements from referring physicians who wished him well. In addition, patients were referred immediately which allowed minimal disruption in his practice.

65 basic marketing tips for health care providers

Despite what some may still think, marketing your group practice doesn't mean using strong-armed, hard-sell tactics. It's as simple as practicing quality medicine, giving your patients good customer service and building a positive brand name identity in your community. Most of all, it means communicating and meeting the needs of your customers.

Remember, there are some simple tips that will be useful in your practice—and help alleviate your concerns about marketing. As noted previously, you may find some or all appropriate for your practice.

Market research

1. Start by finding out who your target audience is, what they want and how they perceive your practice. Gather information from your local Chamber of Commerce, the Census Bureau and other sources.

2. Know your competition—and what they're doing.

3. Survey your current patients to determine what they think about your practice.

Strategic planning

4. If you don't know where you're going, you won't know how to get there. Begin with a well-thought-out strategic marketing plan that's designed to create awareness, project a positive image and increase usage of your services.

5. Don't do anything with which you don't feel comfortable. But do something!

6. Build in a system of tracking—to measure your progress against your plan. Make sure you understand the reasons for any deviation.

7. When your budget is limited, start slow and add programs gradually.

In-office marketing

8. Make your reception area a pleasant, informative place for your patients. Keep

it clean and neat. Provide a small desk with your imprinted stationery and pens—plus a phone for local calls.

9.   Be sure your staff greets each patient by name within 20 seconds of arrival.

10. Provide cold and hot drinks or juice for patients when they must wait. Consider hiring a patient relations hostess to welcome them.

11. In addition to the usual magazines, stock some on health care topics and other less common titles. Make sure they're current issues.

12. Have your office manager arrange for long-lasting flowers in your reception area each week.

13. Place a toy box full of child-safe toys in your reception area. Be sure to include children's books on your shelves. Give children a small puzzle or coloring book imprinted with your practice name to take with them.

14. Keep patients from becoming impatient by having them fill out forms or questionnaires, reviewing educational materials or being pre-screened while they're waiting to be seen by you.

15. Consider developing or purchasing videotapes which patients can view to educate them about specific topics.

Patient communications

16. Prepare and distribute a patient handbook to introduce your practice, explain your office policies and list special services and procedures.

17. Offer free reprints of interesting and informative health care articles or specific procedures or treatments related to your practice.

18. Publish a periodic patient newsletter to provide information about your practice, staff and patients. Also include many photos, case studies and health care news your patients can use. Remember, consistency is more important than frequency—so start with a quarterly or semi-annual issue.

19. Develop a professional-looking, consistent stationery package which includes letterhead, envelope, invoice, business card(s), appointment card, note card and envelope, prescription pad and Rolodex card (if appropriate).

20. Regularly review all materials (such as Yellow Pages and community ads) to assure accuracy and consistency.

21. Have your receptionist give every new patient a copy of your handbook and other policies and procedures with the medical information form.

22. If appropriate, develop a surgery information packet for patients, including pre-op and post-op instructions, along with a comprehensive explanation of what you do and why you recommend follow-up care. Patients are more likely to follow instructions when they understand fully why they're being asked to do them.

23. Install bulletin boards in your exam rooms and ask your staff to post interesting articles on subjects relating to health care or your specialty.

24. Have personalized business cards printed for all your staff. Encourage them to use these cards with patients and everyone else with whom they come in contact.

25. Listen to what your patients ask you. Establish eye contact with them and use their names to show your concern for them.

26. Let your patients know when you've completed a CME course or training in a new technique. Include in your newsletter or send a special "Thought you'd like to know" card.

27. Send a follow-up letter to new patients, thanking them for choosing you and briefly summarizing their diagnosis. Reiterate the importance of follow-up appointments (if appropriate) and regular check-ups.

Customer service

28. Remember that it costs five times as much to acquire a new patient as it does to keep an existing one.

29. Remember that 91 percent of unhappy patients will never visit again, but they will make their dissatisfaction known to at least nine other people. That means, if you turn off one patient, you discourage 10!

30. Let elderly and disabled patients know if you can provide transportation to and from your office.

31. Call patients the day after they've had surgery or an office procedure to see how they're doing. You'll be surprised at the impact it creates.

32. Survey a sample of your patients each year to learn more about their needs, wants and expectations in regard to your services.

33. Periodically, send a brief postage-paid evaluation card/survey to the home of each patient after his or her visit. Use responses to praise outstanding employees and correct any negatives.

34. Have yourself videotaped responding to your 10 most frequently asked questions. It's a great patient-education tool—and it saves time too!

35. Consider creating a Patient Council made up of 10 to 15 typical patients. Bring them together periodically to provide input, recommend improvements and new services to consider.

36. Make it convenient for patients to see you. Set practice hours for evenings and one or two Saturdays a month for people who can't get to your office during weekdays.

37. Personally give every patient your business card. Thank them for choosing you for their care.

38. Have your staff acknowledge all callers and wait for a response before putting them on hold.

39. Ask patients if they understand their diagnosis and/or instructions. Listen to what they tell you.

Referral physicians

40. Report back by phone and be willing to talk about your findings. Referral doctors want to learn from you.

41. Make referrers feel as if they're part of the team—that you'll report to them promptly and you'll send their patients back to them.

42. Send a thorough response—a detailed, diagnostic report—for every referral. Include an executive summary at the beginning of the report.

43. Be available to referring doctors. Set aside a specific time to return calls.

44. Schedule referred patients as quickly as possible. Set aside a block of time each day for this purpose—and let referrers know about it.

45. Copy and send interesting articles about your specialty to present and potential referrers.

46. Hold an annual educational seminar about your specialty. Arrange for CME credits.

47. Work with referring doctors to conduct joint research.

48. Make sure regular referrers know that they are important to you. Stay in touch and thank them regularly with a note or small token gift or invite them to a special event.

49. Thank the staff of referrers by doing something special for one office each month. Send an appropriate token gift to the office or have your staff take their staff to lunch or bring lunch to them.

Internal relations

50. Review all staff policies and procedures regularly.

51. "Recharge batteries" with staff retreats.

52. Make sure your office manager belongs to a national professional organization and encourage him/her to keep up to date and attend their professional/educational meetings.

53. Reward long-time employees with incentives (such as a lapel pin or a restaurant gift certificate).

54. Hire the right staff. Make sure your mission statement is part of their orientation.

55. Have written job descriptions, hold meaningful staff meetings and create an employee handbook.

56. Teach your staff to answer the phone cheerfully and professionally. Write a script that everyone can follow easily.

57. Make sure your staff returns patient phone calls promptly and cheerfully. Don't ever make a patient feel like a nuisance.

58. Empower your staff to make decisions. (Be sure to set up the necessary systems.)

Community relations

59. Build time into your schedule to integrate into the community.

60. Look for opportunities to contract directly with large groups or organizations.

61. Sponsor a Little League (or other) team.

62. Develop an AIDS policy and educate your staff and patients about it.

63. Contact your local, state and national politicians and ask them to keep you up-to-date on any legislation that might affect your practice.

64. Check with industries near your office. Volunteer to contribute health care articles for their monthly newsletters.

65. Make friends with the media.

By following even a few of these tips, you will be miles ahead in your marketing efforts.

Chapter 4

SET: Know Thyself

"There is no more delicate manner to take in hand, nor more dangerous to conduct, nor more doubtful to success, then to step up as a leader in the introduction of changes. For he who innovates will have for his enemies all those who are well-off under the existing order of things, and only lukewarm supporters and those who might be better off under the new."

—Niccolo Machiavelli

To succeed in health care today, you must know yourself—and your practice. How do you do that? Where do you begin?

First, you have to decide what you stand for, what you represent. You must clearly understand, commit to and communicate your:

- Mission;
- Vision;
- Code of ethics;
- Commitment to quality; and
- Accountability.

In addition, you have to know exactly where your practice stands in the marketplace and where you want it to go. And you must make sure that every employee you hire understands and shares your vision and commitment.

This is the simple concept that forms the basis of all marketing. Undoubtedly, that's why it is subscribed to by every major company, including Walt Disney World, Darden Restaurants, Microsoft, Ritz Carlton and USA Today. They all have a crystal-clear vision of who they are and where they want to go.

Knowing who you are grows out of a comprehensive—internal and external—assessment of your practice. And, such an assessment begins with knowing your mission. Everything you do should form a concentric circle around that mission.

Your mission is a statement which describes why your organization exists, what services and/or products it offers and to whom the service and products are offered. It's an expression of your values, goals and purpose—a code of conduct for your practice. For example, it should answer the following questions:

- What business are you in?
- Why do you exist?
- Who do you serve?
- Where are you headed?

The best way to create a practice mission statement is to begin by asking the entire staff to contribute what they consider to be the values, goals and purpose of the practice. As an exercise, ask everyone to complete the following statement:

> The mission of our practice is to _____.

Take all the information you've gathered and compile it into a few (two to eight) sentences that comprise a comprehensive expression of the essence of your practice. If you've done it honestly and completely, you have a mission statement that will guide your practice toward success. A later chapter will show several examples.

You also must clearly understand and state your vision. This is a declaration of the future state of your organization—the future you want to create for your practice. It's based on reasonable beliefs as to what is worthwhile, challenging and inspirational.

In Chapter 6, you'll find several examples of vision statements of national organizations that you'll recognize. Can your practice model after these?

Once you've compiled your mission and vision statements, identify and commit to paper the values that support them. Although this list is not complete, you may find the following characteristics helpful as you think about values:

- Courtesy;
- Accountability;
- Efficiency;
- Respect;
- Honesty;
- Profitability;

- Productivity;
- Loyalty;
- Accuracy;
- Excellence;
- Teamwork;
- Dependability;
- Commitment;
- Dedication; and
- Attitude.

The core values of your group are easily understood statements which describe how your group behaves while accomplishing its mission and vision. They set your standards of excellence and reflect the high ideals of your group. They are what inspires enthusiasm and encourages commitment to your mission.

Values are the qualities that you prize or believe have worth for their own sake, such as honesty, accountability, commitment, integrity, teamwork, caring, efficiency, sympathy, empathy, training and patient orientation. Research shows that group practices which formalize their value system, integrate it into their overall daily operations—and communicate it to all employees—overwhelmingly outperform practices that do not. Staff who work for management that consistently models positive values are much more likely to exert the added effort needed to ensure that patients receive certain and superior quality service.

For more information on this subject, I highly recommend that you take a look at MGMA's 1999 publication, *Performance and Practices of Successful Medical Groups*. Its authors point out several key points about the importance of instilling values in today's group practices. For example, on page 6, as the report discusses culture building, it says, "Many groups are keenly aware that continued success depends on inculcating positive group values in new physicians."

As a health care professional today, you obviously realize that the market is rapidly moving from a productivity system to a capitated system. You understand that the Rubik's Cube has been completely turned—360 degrees.

What does this mean? Why is it important?

It's valuable because it gives you the chance to look at things differently—to break new ground, rather than do things as they've always been done. It gives you an opportunity to differentiate your practice from the rest of the pack.

Let's look at an example. Everyone knows that when you're paid fee-for-service, you're paid on productivity. You want to see many patients, as often as you can, because that is in your best financial interest.

However, within a capitated system, as you know, your goal is to see patients no more than is necessary. After all, you get paid only a set fee per patient per month, not per visit. This gives you an opportunity (even a responsibility) to teach yourself, your staff and your patients how and when to use your practice appropriately and usefully.

Obviously, you want patients to visit your practice when they really need to come. And when they do come, you want to educate them about their disease, when to use your practice, how to use it, and how to be the most comfortable in their efforts to have a successful outcome. If you work closely with them, you can keep them from using the system unnecessarily and from using unnecessary resources.

As your practice gains knowledge and implements more efficient ways to manage disease, you can reduce health care resource utilization while still achieving a satisfactory outcome. Rather than deny patient care, you'll look at each situation in terms of what is in the best interest of the patient.

As you recognize how to do that, you will be able to communicate this to your staff as well as to your employer customers. Remember, it's important that you share your vision with them as well as with managed care insurers, who have an interest in knowing about groups which consciously practice efficiently, effectively and with a service mentality.

At the same time, you should look at the value-added factors that exist within your practice. "Value-added" includes all the attributes that differentiate your practice from others, along with the benefits from doing business with your practice and anything else that makes your practice special.

You can view value-added as a gift. You put the present in a box. Everything else is added value. The wrapping paper, the bow and the note card all contribute to making the present different and more highly valued by the recipient.

Look at your practice in the same way. Value-added is all around us. It may be difficult to describe because it's probably everything you take for granted. Begin to ask your staff, your physicians and yourself what makes your practice different. Take a minute to absorb all the information and compile it for your value-added differentiation statement.

Assessing your practice

Next, assess your practice with an eye toward finding ways to maintain and increase your market share. Begin by examining your practice's SWOT (strengths, weaknesses, opportunities and threats) and defining your goals. This will allow you to prioritize your marketing challenges.

As you assess your community, identify major employers and primary referrers, as well as practices positioned as gatekeepers. Also, list existing managed care plans, managed care plans that are entering the community, Medicaid HMOs and Medicare HMOs.

When conducting an internal managed care assessment, look at your contracts, affiliations, fee schedules, payer mix, revenues and procedural fees. Evaluate capitated contracts and their significance within your practice. When you do an external managed care assessment, look at enrollment, products, major customers, new initiatives, market share and your competitors.

Managed Care Assessment

At all times, keep in mind that the relationships of the future are being built today. And with so many consolidations taking place, the person you work with at one organization today may very well be the same one you'll work with at a different organization tomorrow!

Another part of your assessment is to identify your customers so you can develop and implement appropriate marketing strategies which will meet their needs. As noted in Chapter 2, they most likely will be patients, referring physicians, managed care companies, employers, and integrated delivery systems.

As you are assessing, research what your patients want. The FACT organization, a byproduct of the Jackson Hole Group, learned this about patient desires. Patients want their physicians to:
- Honor their values and preferences;
- Respect them as persons;
- Communicate clearly;
- Give them power;
- Heal them as whole persons;
- Coordinate across complexity of care; and
- Change our relationship from autocratic to partner.

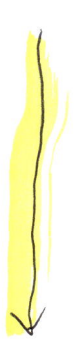

Having learned that, you can implement the following marketing strategies:
- Treat patients as guests;
- Educate patients via technology;

- Conduct patient surveys;
- Create database for mailings;
- Provide patients with educational information;
- Call selected patients following their visit;
- Empower all staff to be personable and personal and accountable; and
- Address your patients with appropriate respect.

As you conduct your assessment, you also should identify referral physician needs. These include but are not limited to:

- Giving patients quality care;
- Having patients referred back for care;
- Receiving prompt informative reports;
- Having referred patients scheduled promptly; and
- Having your practice be accountable.

This allows you to implement the following strategies:

- Create a database of your referral physicians;
- Keep referrers informed and involved;
- Make it easy for referrers to reach you;
- Offer a dedicated referral phone line;
- Organize a think-tank with referrers for difficult cases;
- Develop measurable marketing activities; and
- Provide clinical newsletters or mailings.

Again, in your assessment, you're going to be looking at managed care needs. Among other things these customers want cost-effectiveness, geographic access, best-demonstrated practices, payer-friendly physicians, and your support at re-credentialing time.

To address these needs, your group might want to consider implementing the following marketing strategies:

- Share your UR outcomes;
- Hold personal meetings twice year;
- Communicate practice differentiation;
- Track patients and revenues;
- Gain access to their employers;
- Communicate everything in writing;
- Share cost-reduction strategies;
- Get to know administrative personnel; and
- Obtain direct marketing approval via your contract.

Finally, as you assess the wants and need of employers, you'll learn that their top priorities are quality, access and pricing. Value purchasing is also important to them, and frequently, they are willing to develop relationships with providers.

Having this knowledge will allow you to implement the following strategies:
* Keep employers updated;
* Make contact with new employers;
* Get to know the benefits manager;
* Create database for mailings;
* Write articles for company newsletters;
* Invite employers to lunch and to tour your practice; and
* Correspond via physician letter or newsletter.

If you have previously conducted these assessments, it's a good idea to take another look periodically. When you do, be sure to step back and be very objective. Evaluate your existing goals to be sure they are still current and that they address what you want for your future. Examine your mission statement to determine if it's still valid, and enumerate the value-added characteristics that differentiate your practice from your competitors. Make sure that your Management Information System (MIS) has adequate capability to handle the important operational issues that will arise as your practice matures. Finally, as is emphasized throughout this book, you must be very sensitive to customer service issues.

Figure 4-a

Practice assessment features

SWOT's

When assessing your practice, you may want to consider some of the following typical characteristics of a subspecialty practice.

STRENGTHS:
* Minimal competition (because of creative positioning);
* Good geographic location;
* Strong work ethic;
* Willingness to change;
* Practice sub-specialization;
* Strong practice administrator;
* Strategic recruiting process; and
* Belief in marketing.

WEAKNESSES:

- Lack of a group mentality;
- Lack of vision;
- Group apathy;
- Inability to make decisions;
- Large size (causing a perception of a factory or bureaucratic mentality);
- Lack of strong leadership;
- Minimal market share; and
- Lack of marketing.

THREATS:

- Merger of other specialty groups within the region;
- National specialty management company in a relationship with local managed care plans impacting our business;
- Exclusion from physician-developed networks;
- Failure to develop MIS compromises our ability to compete with other groups who have invested in MIS; and   *Management Information System*
- Patients are seeking treatment at national care centers outside the community due to the ease of doing research on the Internet.

OPPORTUNITIES:

- Join or be a developmental leader in a specialty network;
- Develop a physician panel to do provider relations with the local health care coalition;
- Maximize on the health systems strategy to re-energize relations with their medical staff;
- Develop an equity position in a specialty hospital or surgical center;
- Contract to provide services in outlying areas via the use of technology; and
- Re-locate an existing office with declining census to an area of high residential and commercial growth.

VALUE-ADDED DIFFERENTIATION:

- Physician credentials;
- Specially credentialed staff;
- Location or geographic distribution of office sites;
- Operational systems;
- MIS systems;
- Practice capabilities;
- Willingness to accept risk;

- Global pricing; and
- Focus on building relationships with payers and employers.

Figure 4-b

Self-assessment guidelines

- Know who you are;
- Know what you want;
- Know your customers;
- Know what your customers want;
- Know your group and its capabilities;
- Have a marketing plan;
- Know what legal constraints there on marketing and structure your plan accordingly;
- Understand that marketing is an evolution of behaviors and layers of activities;
- Write down specific goals;
- Develop basic communication tools;
- Build your brand;
- Hold a strategic retreat;
- Support your internal staff and empower them;
- Understand media relations and use the media as a resource;
- Put yourself in a mind-set to lead in your community;
- Recognize the power of customer service;
- Recognize that patients are number one and have a great deal of power; and
- Do it well, even if you cannot do it all.

Figure 4-c

Sample goals and strategies worksheet

(Note: This worksheet is used successfully by an orthopaedic practice, but is applicable for any type of practice.)

- Goal #1: To enhance positive relations with our referral physicians:
    - Strategy #1: Create a database for effective communication; and
    - Strategy #2 Initiate a referral physician survey.

- Goal # 2: To provide patient education about our practice's physicians, products and services to our patients:
    - Strategy #1: Create a directory of practice physicians and services;
    - Strategy #2: Create a display in our reception area; and
    - Strategy #3: Develop a fact sheet to use at expos.

- Goals #3: To educate/train our internal staff to provide excellent customer service:
    - Strategy #1 Send staff to customer relations workshops;
    - Strategy #2: Role-play responses to patient complaints; and
    - Strategy #3: Hold an annual staff retreat.

- Goal #4: To serve as a liaison with our local sports team:
    - Strategy #1 Participate in mutual marketing;
    - Strategy #2: Create a sports "wall of fame" in patient areas; and
    - Strategy #3 Participate in fan appreciation day.

- Goal #5: To build and maintain positive image with our local community through targeted health expos:
    - Strategy #1 Research employer-based health expos;
    - Strategy #2: Participate in local golf expo; and
    - Strategy #3 Participate in expos that attract student athletes.

Figure 4-d
Setting goals

Goals without plans are a dream. So, as you think about your customers, think about their needs. Then, set your own group goals to meet those needs. An easy exercise is to:

- List your goals;
- Look at them every day of your life;
- Share your professional goals with your staff; and
- Involve your staff with the top three goals of the practice.

Remember, there is no such thing as an unrealistic goal—just an unrealistic timetable.

Figure 4-e
Marketing questionnaire

Here are some important questions that should be asked of practice administrators and physicians as a part of a practice assessment.

Focus on your practice

1. What are your business objectives?

2. What are your strengths? What are the strengths of your practice?

3. What are your weaknesses? What are the weaknesses of your practice?

4. What do you see as the threats to your practice?

5. What do you see as the opportunities for your practice?

6. What factors are critical to your future?

7. What has contributed to your success to date?

8. What do you see as your most critical marketing needs? Please list them in order of priority.

9. Do you have regular meetings with your staff? How often? What is discussed?

Is your staff paid overtime to stay for such meetings?

Services offered

1. What services do you presently offer?

2. What kinds of cases do you see most often? Least often?

3. How has your caseload changed over the past year?

4. Do you think it is likely to change over the coming year?

5. Which of your regular procedures are the most cost effective?

6. Which procedures that you enjoy doing provide the highest profit margin?

7. Which of your regular procedures can be done on an outpatient basis?

8. Do you see the need to become involved in an outpatient surgical facility?

9. Would this be a hospital-sponsored facility, a joint venture with other physicians or owned wholly by your practice?

10. Would you consider becoming a member of a large group practice?

Patients

1. From what geographic areas do your present patients come?

2. From what age and socioeconomic groups?

3. Is your patient mix changing? How?

4. How are new patients currently entering your practice?

5. What reason do patients give for leaving your practice?

6. What attitudes do patients show toward your practice?

7. Do you feel your present patients are aware of ALL the services you offer?

8. What kinds of patients do you wish to attract to your practice?

9. Explain your scheduling plan for new patient visits, surgical visits, medical treatment visits, and post-op visits.

10. List three ways you currently help patients understand and deal with your fees.

11. Suggest three ways you could improve upon the previous three.

12. What are the policies and coverage extents of third-party insurers in your area?

Local physicians

1. Which physicians currently refer to your practice? Why?

2. Which physicians do not? Why?

3. How familiar are area physicians with the services offered by your practice?

4. How do you welcome new physicians into your community?

5. Do you have a plan to meet informally with referring doctors or new physicians in the community? Please explain that plan.

6. Do you see a need to network with potential referring doctors? Do you know how to network?

7. What opportunities do you have for referring patients to family practice or internal medicine physicians? How often? To whom do you refer under these circumstances?

8. Are you involved in the medical education of potential referring doctors?

9. How do you identify referral sources and make contact with them, both physicians and patients?

10. Do you have a referral reference system that identifies the referring patient or physician, the referring physician's specialty, address or location, referring patient's insurance carrier, and frequency of referrals?

11. What medical board affiliations do you hold? Which ones are recognized as accredited specialty boards by those other than board members?

12. Can you see yourself as a catalyst in organizing leading physicians to develop a physician network?

13. What percentage of your community is involved in managed care plans?

14. In which managed care plans and/or PPOs do you participate?

15. Do you network with other physicians on hospital committees, in community organizations, or in board-appointed positions? Please identify these.

Local community

1. What is the average family composition in your community?

2. What is the projected population growth of your community?

3. Do you think the present population mix will change? How?

4. What are the health care patterns utilized in your community? How much Medicaid? Medicare? Managed care? CHAMPUS? Fee-for-service?

5. Do you feel your community is aware of your practice and the services it offers?

6. To what community organizations do you belong?

7. What community events do you sponsor as an organization?

Your competition

1. How many physicians are there in your specialty?

2. How many are there in other specialties that may compete for your patients?

3. How many ambulatory care centers are there that compete with you?

4. What other organizations or individuals represent serious competition?

5. What services do you have in common with your competition?

6. How could you improve them to offer better quality than your competition?

7. What services do you offer that your competition does not?

8. In what ways do you plan to differentiate, expand and diversify your service offerings to either maintain or increase your market share to combat increasing competition over the next two to five years?

Expanding services to meet changing patient needs

1. List three ways you are now meeting the special needs of specific patient groups.

2. Suggest three ways you think you could expand the services presently offered by your practice.

3. At what hospitals do you currently have privileges?

4. If you were going to expand your practice, where would your next office be located? Why?

5. What are your current office hours? Have you expanded your hours to accommodate the working population? If not, why?

Increasing visibility and promoting services to patients

1. List three ways you are currently promoting your practice and its services.

2. Suggest three ways you could make your practice more visible to prospective patients.

3. What TV, radio and print exposure have you received? Who handled contacts with the media? Did you have any noticeable results?

4. In which editions of the Yellow Pages do you currently advertise? Which areas do they cover?

5. Have you ever invited people from hospital PR departments to tour your office and job-shadow you?

6. Have you ever scheduled appointments with hospital CEOs to explain your practice goals?

7. Identify your social involvement in charities, arts councils, and other settings where potential referring physicians or patients are involved.

8. In what professional and social organizations do you maintain memberships? Are you active in them?

9. How do you feel about letting the media job-shadow you?

10. Do you write and publish articles? How often? Where?

Creating satisfied, loyal patients who will refer others

1. Apart from treatment itself, list three ways you are working to create satisfied patients.

2. Suggest three ways you might further enhance your patients' overal satisfaction.

Look to the future

1. If your group were an unparalleled success—the best group of its type in the world—what would it look like?

2. Look at the leader of the group and the management team that supports the leader. What are their greatest strengths?

3. What suggestions would you offer the leader that would help him/her become an even more effective leader?

4. What outcomes do you hope to achieve as you work together?

5. Identify the five most important issues your group needs to address in the next three years in order to fulfill your mission and achieve your vision.

6. Identify where your group should be focusing its energy and resources to have the greatest impact.

7. Keeping in mind that strategic goals need to be specific enough to be measured and represent an end result which you can achieve in three years, develop these springboards:
   • What if...?
   • I wish we....
   • How would I/we...?

8. Please answer the following questions for the year 2003:
   • How do you work with your stakeholders?
   • How do you produce value for them?
   • What is your group's greatest legacy?
   • What would the community lose if your group ceased to exist?

9. Please answer the following questions for the year 2003:
   • What fundamental needs is your group fulfilling for your customers?
   • How have you surpassed your competition?
   • What are your products and services?
   • What else is your group known for?
   • Who are the stakeholders of the practice you've created?

10. Why is it important to articulate values for your group? Because they (add others which apply):
   • Guide day-to-day decisions;
   • Create group culture;
   • Help screen potential employees and orient new employees; and
   • Hold each other accountable.

11. Can your group be successful at achieving the goals it has set?

12. Is there sufficient capital to fund those strategies?

13. Does your organization have the infrastructure necessary to support the people, processes, and technology in order to implement its strategies?

14. If your group implements its plan, will it have a positive impact on the group's position and form a platform for future growth?

15. How will the implementation of strategies affect the following?
    - Market position;
    - Leadership role;
    - Financial position and economic goals; and
    - Group culture.

Internet communications

1. Do you have a practice Web page?

2. How often is it updated? By whom?

3. Does it reflect new products and services?

4. Does your medical practice have a chat room?

5. Do you educate patients to use the chat room to get hints on self-help shortcuts?

6. Do you encourage your patients to e-mail questions for their physician or other clinical support help?

7. Do you communicate about health talks offered throughout the year on your Web page?

8. Does your staff communicate with patients via e-mail?

Commitment

1. What will you do to help your group accomplish these goals, fulfill its mission and achieve its vision?

Chapter **5**

Empowering and Supporting Internal Staff

"If you can't change the facts, try bending your attitude."
—George Eliot, 19th-century English novelist

In the area of staff empowerment, few people are more experienced than my colleague Dan Frankel, Ph.D. I met Dr. Frankel professionally several years ago and was impressed by the insight and expertise he provided for a mutual client. Having worked with him since then on numerous occasions, I asked him to contribute his expertise to this chapter.

Dr. Frankel is a principal of Martin/Frankel Associates, which specializes in building organizational effectiveness. His expertise includes change management and individual and team-based executive development. He has worked with small to large Fortune 100 privately-held and publicly-traded companies. He also consults with regional medical alliances and small group practices experiencing business transition. The following discussion synthesizes many of his thoughts that are applicable to medical practices.

The engaged organization: A case for change

Most physicians are motivated self-directed people who care deeply about their patients and take their responsibility for the medical well-being of their patients very seriously. Most work hard and believe they give much of themselves and of their families to be available to their patients. They know that this is part of the price they have to pay to experience the pride and excitement of practicing medicine.

In return, most physicians expect—even if the understanding is only an implicit contract—that they will be provided full and unquestioned control of patient care. They expect to be allowed to remain undistracted by any consideration other than what they believe is appropriate patient care. Most believe the objective of the medical practice should be to do anything and everything to maximize the physician's patient care.

Traditionally, the organizational model of the medical practice has involved the physician's giving orders that others execute in order to comply with the demands of authority. In today's world, of course, the requirements of a successful private practice conflict with such expectations. It just won't work that way anymore.

Therefore, the structure and management of private medical practice has to evolve. Today, physicians not only have to maintain responsibility for their individual actions, they also must keep in mind the overall functioning of the practice. Individual roles must be subordinated to a larger entity. Delegation and accommodation become requisites that no longer are negotiable. Expertise may not always dictate which activities accrue the most benefit to the practice.

The practice may best rationalize the role even of a highly skilled physician by having that doctor devote a significant part of his/her work effort to activities, such as marketing and new business development. In short, today's medical practices have to understand that they are professional services firms.

Many organizations—particularly large corporations in the private sector—have already had to confront the need to change. Corporations were forced to recognize that in an increasingly competitive marketplace, those who figure out how to reduce and minimize the cost of doing business—the cost of business transactions—could quickly seize a competitive advantage that affords either greater profit or, because of reduced price to the consumer, an increased market share.

Service-based industries such as medicine need to pay attention to these issues and lessons. Reimbursement sources consistently pay less for specific services and procedures. In order to survive and compete in this environment, medical practices are merging and growing in size.

Conventional wisdom not withstanding, larger organizations rarely are more cost efficient than smaller organizations. Thus, the growing medical practice has to pay even greater attention to the way business is conducted or, paradoxically, the presumed benefits of size will only accrue on the liability side of the ledger.

What the large corporation can teach even the small- to middle-sized private practice is that efficiency is achieved by creating a different type of organization—one that engages the talents of all the individuals who contribute to the organization.

Normal reactions to the case for change

The need for change in the organization and management of the medical practice may be obvious. Still, it is important to note that no matter how vigorous the endorsement of change by the physician, the effort to implement change will be accompanied by resistance.

Change is not just movement to improved or better circumstances. Change involves giving up—giving up of identity, roles, status and competencies. Little surprise that even in the business sector, more than half of the time change initiatives fail.

Typically, initial resistance to change expresses itself in denial. The successful physician insists that continued professionalism, expertise and availability should be all it takes to sustain success. Being a good doctor should be enough for patients to be referred and to find satisfaction. It isn't. A successful physician has to be part of an organization, and his/her individual skills simply aren't enough.

It truly is the practice and not the individual physician that defines success. And, the successful practice must place priority on the organization and the marketing of the organization—a far cry from patients on their own seeking out the expertise of the talented outstanding doctor.

Requirements for change

How can the efficiency of the business management of the growing medical practice be increased? What makes employees "own" the challenges of improving the efficiencies of doing business and projecting the desired behaviors toward the different external and internal constituencies/clients the business contacts?

The first step is a vision, oftentimes a "motherhood and apple pie" statement that nonetheless can build pride and reassure employees that their work has meaning and integrity. The vision—making all our patients feel as if they were family—can have a difficult to obtain or even unobtainable quality, but this sets a tone for the enterprise. It reminds us why we are doing what we are doing.

Sometimes, vision statements are greeted with skepticism. Unfortunately, such feelings often are legitimate. For example, consider the commercial airline which hangs a banner stating its primary commitment to its people. At the same time, the poor state of the company's customer service makes it difficult to believe this is an authentic reflection of the way it really does business. In those circumstances, will anyone believe the vision statement is sincere?

The point is not that visions are meaningless mottoes. The point is that they have to be authentic statements of the practice's commitments. The practice has to mean what it says and then manage itself in a manner that is congruent with its promises.

Business practices have to match the promises. If they don't, we are, in effect, teaching others that we lie, that we say one thing but really mean and do another. If this is the implicit policy lesson a practice is teaching its employees, how will they act when providing service to its customers? Wittingly or unwittingly, the practice provides the message that establishes the norm for its people.

An authentic vision statement represents a deliberate and considered effort to make sure we can articulate what we want to be and that we understand the implications of that message. We need to make sure we know what, in fact, we are communicating to our employees. In addition, we must make sure that is how we want to characterize the business dealings of the members of the organization, both internally and externally.

Vision statements clearly are not enough on their own to set a practical direction to the organization. A vision statement has to be translated into goals, into ways people will work together to meet the needs of the different customers; e.g. patients, referral sources, vendors, employees, etc. In effect, the leadership of the practice has to be able to lay out what the objective is—the practice that provides rapid, accurate and thoughtful results to referral sources and treats patients with dignity and a sense of concern and understanding for the frightening, intimidating and anxious experience they are going through—and a "theory" of how this is to be achieved.

This is not unlike what is referred to in the commercial world as creating a brand. People in the Northwest know what Nordstrom stands for—they know that customer service will be the priority for anyone they deal with in the organization. Nordstrom commits itself to customer service and communicates that commitment downstream as the guiding principle for all employees. In simple terms, the vision with its operational goals helps the entire organization focus on the same priorities.

So where's the profit? Even a medical practice that is committed to the care of the patients requires profit, if only to remain in business. Non-profit status is not the desired outcome for most providers. Many businesses today take the risk of assuming that profit is the outcome of delivering a service successfully.

If you really do a good job of delivering a service that meets the needs of the market in a cost-effective way, profit will follow. It is a metric for how well the business is meeting its objectives. Profit is not being ignored, but it is not usually the only—or even the major reason—for the existence of the practice. If it is, then it should be so recognized and all business practices should proceed accordingly.

Outcomes of the engaged organization— employees and patients

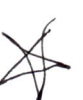

There is a great interdependence between the way employees feel about work and the way others experience the practice. Most of the interaction between patient and practice, for example, involves support personnel.

The values that support personnel project in their behavior and treatment of patients, as well as other customers of the practice, usually reflect the values they learn through their treatment by the practice. They will respect the dignity of others only if they feel their dignity is respected as well. It all works together.

If billing personnel know that their personal concerns, such as compensation, will be treated with respect by human resources personnel, they are more likely to respond in a friendly and understanding manner to patients' billing questions. This, in turn, is likely to increase loyalty to the practice by each of the customers who interact with it. It also is likely to increase efficiencies, because employees who understand the practice remain with the practice. Work is more likely to be accurate, and the direct and indirect costs of recruiting are minimized.

As mentioned previously, traditional medical practice management has been highly controlling of employees. Indeed, it has been rather like the military, deploying a "command and control" method of supervision, starting with the main physician and moving downstream to the head nurse and office manager.

Unfortunately, the pride of participation in an organization like the Marines often does not characterize employment in the private sector. When people are treated as if they can't think on their own or take the initiative, not surprisingly, those who remain conform to that very expectation.

Their focus will be on avoiding the mistake and doing things the way they've been told and the way things always have been done—no matter how reasonable or unreasonable. There is little or no incentive to contribute to an improved way of executing tasks. But there is a heightened likelihood that the resentment and anger over not being valued gets played out with those who come into contact with the business.

Employees are more likely to embrace ownership if they understand what the objective of the enterprise is and how their job fits into it, if they feel achievements are rewarded more than errors punished. They will embrace ownership if management is based more on the responsible actions of the majority, rather than the inadequacies of the minority.

This is not abdication—it is not allowing the insane to run the asylum. It does, however, admit reality—that bosses rarely really dictate what employees do. In fact, employees usually decide implicitly the tasks to which they will devote most of their time. A strike by the pilots of American Airlines in 1999 is a good example of this. Pilots exercised their "right" to be sick and stay home as well their right not to fly overtime. Indeed, their insistence on doing things the way they had negotiated with management—that is, compliance with their labor contract that frees them from having to work overtime—imposed major schedule disruption and financial loss on the airline.

Assuming proper selection, ownership and the subsequent self-direction of employees will occur if:
- They understand the direction of the enterprise;
- They are given proper preparation;
- They are given support for developing overlapping processes with other team members;
- They are held accountable for clearly defined outcomes or deliverables both as individuals and in teams; and
- There is proper recognition for performance that is congruent with expectations and demands.

If the objectives of the organization and the ways it will operate are clear enough, it will be readily possible to resist compromising accountabilities. All of this, of course, assumes a particular theory of human psychology, namely, that most people like to feel competent and valued and experience a sense of belonging. If they do, they will respond positively.

This new type of organizational structure often is referred to as "empowered." In fact, all too often, empowerment means that subordinates are supposed to figure out what the boss wants and how the boss wants it done without the boss' providing much support. In effect, it means the subordinate has to take responsibility for being accountable for doing more with less.

Authentic empowerment, on the other hand, depends on the opportunity for trust— an absence of fear. It depends on a psychological frame of mind. Employees must believe that authority and responsibility come from within themselves.

Empowerment can have an arrogant and patronizing connotation. It can imply that from above comes the opportunity for people to create visions of the way they would like things to be and how they would make that happen.

This notion of empowerment implies that employees work in an environment where power—ultimately compensation, benefits and even job security—is handled capriciously and depends upon figuring out what pleases authority. Empowerment all too readily can become a contradiction in terms. What the healthy medical practice, in fact, should seek is the engagement and initiative of autonomous people who are thinking out ways in which they can contribute to the practice's vision and goals.

Today's engaged organization is not beyond the capability of any small- to mid-size medical practice. It simply requires a recognition that the efficiency and effectiveness of an organization facilitates the efficiency and effectiveness of the medical practitioner. An engaged organization, ironically, allows the physician to focus on what he/she has learned and wishes to provide. The engaged organization reflects an intense, highly thoughtful, honest—and yes, time-consuming—"front-end," but continuing effort to articulate a specific description of the contribution that all employees can make to the meaningfulness of treating human beings who are ill.

Figure 5-a

Tell-tale signs of resistance to change

- *Denial*—insisting that you can continue to do things the way you used to;
- *Avoidance*—finding reasons why you can't implement different ways of functioning even though you claim you accept the need for change;
- *Rationalization*—finding reasons to have to think things through more carefully, engage in more analysis in effect only to defer change;
- *Abdication*—hoping the white knight will come by—looking for someone else to fix things while you continue to operate as you did in the past; and
- *Paralysis*—feeling overwhelmed and depressed, not knowing what to do, feeling hopeless and just wanting to give up.

Figure 5-b

Steps to creating the engaged organization

1. Development and articulation of the vision—motherhood and apple pie.

2. Definition of the business(es) and strategies that will be deployed to create and sustain that business(es)—the mission.

3. Communication of the vision and mission.

4. Identification of vision and mission for each department by the employees who manage that department.

5. Communication of those visions and missions within departments.

6. Development of standards—management commitments to all constituencies that will be dealt with; e.g. patients, referral sources, reimbursement sources, vendors—that are congruent with the missions.

7. Measurement of outcomes—including profitability—that reflect the mission

8. Evaluation of successes and failures—effort at continuous improvement.

9. Uncompromising insistence on meeting the standards agreed upon in the mission.

Note: Execution of these steps is time-consuming and can seem vague and nonproductive. When implemented well, they clearly lay out what we are here to do, how we are going to do it and how we will hold ourselves accountable. This forces a level of integrity, wholeness, congruity, and coherence—upon the organization that means we have to be truly honest about why we are in business and what we are after.

Figure 5-c

Teamwork

Teamwork goes hand-in-hand with empowerment to play a major part of the success of a medical practice. It is your team that will allow your practice to live its vision, meet its goals and accomplish its mission.

We frequently talk about teamwork as it relates to your practice staff. Actually, the relations you have with referring physicians are team-oriented as well. Relationships between physicians traditionally are many years old. Physicians are used to these kinds of relationships. When you think about how you team with a referring physician in the broadest sense of the term, you think about having complete communications, providing appropriate patient care, realizing that for both, a few of the stakes are higher now.

It's very important to build on these relationships. You both benefit when you share utilization protocols. It matters that you can demonstrate quality assurance and document cost-effective care.

Here is an old example of teamwork that I learned while working on a group project. It was shared with the group but sadly listed no author.

- When geese fly in formation, they travel about 70 percent faster than when they fly alone.
- Geese share leadership. When the lead goose tires, he/she rotates back into the "V," and another flies forward to become a leader.
- Geese keep company with the fallen. When a sick or weak goose falls out of flight formation, at least one other goose joins to help and protect.
- By being part of a team, you too can accomplish much more, much faster. Words of encouragement and support (honking from behind) will help inspire you and energize those on the front lines—helping them keep pace in spite of the day-to-day pressures and fatigue.
- And finally, show compassion and an active caring for your fellow man—a member of the ultimate team: "mankind." The next time you see a formation of geese, remember that it is a reward, a challenge and a privilege to be a contributing member of a team.

Figure 5-d

Successful team profile

- The ability to work together;
- A vision;
- Clear and simple objectives;
- Trust among the team;
- A variety of disciplines represented;
- Available resources;
- An openness in idea sharing;
- Common sense;
- Risk takers;
- Good communicators;
- Flexibility;
- A sense of humor and fun;
- Self-confidence;
- Passion; and
- A belief in the organization.

Figure 5-e

Signs of a healthy team

- **Dynamic vision/focus on future not on past**
  - A recognition that things change and the past cannot be relied upon when establishing policies for the future. Team members also must let go of past feelings and seek a way of working with others to obtain a future.

- **Intentional communication**
  - A commitment to communicate with all others who believe they should be included.

- **Constructive conflict resolution**
  - Disagreement is healthy and avoids unthinking consensus. Management of conflict is critical.

- **Patience with process of change**
    - Team members have to understand that change takes t me and the issues that guide change need to be revisited repeatedly.

- **Integrity/absence of deception**
    - Even if people don't have to volunteer their understanding of truth to everyone all the time, efforts must be made to act in ways that are congruent with articulated values and principles for the workplace.

Cleveland Clinic Testimonial

Richard Harris has renal cell cancer, a chronic difficult disease. This disease does not respond to chemotherapy or radiation therapy. Instead, as lesions are identified on either CT Scan or MRI, they are surgically removed. Harris has had surgery in his local community hospital, as well as at a prestigious Boston academic medical center.

He was not unhappy with the care he received at either place. But when his disease re-occurred again in 1998, he began to research which institution had focused expertise in renal cell cancer. This time, the disease was once again in his lungs and also in his only remaining kidney. His research directed him to the Cleveland Clinic Foundation.

Once he was accepted as a patient, he was into a 12-month relationship. It began with developing a relationship with a CCF oncologist who is very active in the National Kidney Cancer Foundation and in ongoing clinical trials for renal cell disease. The oncologist laid out the options for Harris. It would be important to surgically remove the lesions from his lungs and his kidney. All along the way, as they cared for his disease, CT Scans would be done to evaluate the progression of the disease.

Harris lives in Florida, not in Ohio. This made communication between the Clinic and his household very important. Once he made his initial visit to the surgeon and it was determined that his lung surgery would precede the kidney surgery, Harris was presented with the schedule relating to his admission. When he recovered from lung surgery, he would be immediately scheduled for kidney surgery.

Harris found a number of things relating to his hospitalizations quite impressive. The Clinic sent his schedule for diagnostic testing, physician appointments and admission two weeks before his visit. He found something comfortable about knowing what was going to happen to him on his visit.

When he arrived for his first appointment of the morning, he never had to provide anything other than his insurance card, even though he was from out-of-state. And he never had to show that card other than once at the beginning of the day.

He always felt that he was expected at each of the appointment areas. He was greeted by name and informed how long he would wait before being taken for each appointment. He found each department always on schedule, no matter what time or day he was there. In fact, he noticed a sign posted in every reception area in which he waited. It said, "If you have been waiting longer than 15 minutes, please notify our receptionist." Harris never waited that long to be called for a scheduled appointment. It was that way every visit, every time. He wondered why his physicians at home couldn't do the same thing, particularly when their offices seemed far less busy.

On a follow-up visit after Harris's second surgery, the CT Scan showed that his disease was again progressing. His oncologist offered him some options. Together, they made a decision for Harris to enter a research clinical trial for patients with renal cell cancer. It was quite a difficult time for Harris. He realized that his cancer was a chronic disease. He became aware that surgery was not going to solve his problem this time. He realized he had some big decisions to make.

Returning to Florida, Harris discussed his options with his family, spoke with his employer, talked to his insurer and called back to his oncologist in Cleveland. He agreed to enter the clinical trial even though it meant staying in Cleveland for an entire month. Laura, the research nurse who Harris had met during a brief introduction, asked him if he had an e-mail address. No one had asked that before. He provided her with his address and from that moment on, another relationship was born. The e-mails went something like this.

Subject: Appt schedule
Date: Fri, 12 Feb 1999 16:09:48 -0500
From: Laura, RN@cc.ccf.org
To: RHarris@trock.com

Hope your trip home went okay. I have the appointment schedule for Feb 19, 20, and 22 for you. The schedule will be mailed to you, but I wanted you to have it ASAP. Do I need to fax a script for the bone scan to you?

Feb 19
12:00 Lab
12:15 Laura
1:00 EKG
1:45 DLCO
3:00 MUGA
4:30 CXR

Feb 20
10:30 CT Scan

Feb 22
8:00 Dr. Walsh and Laura
Start treatment

Let me know if you have any other questions, or things I can do to help.
Laura

This was the beginning of an e-mail relationship that empowered Harris to prepare himself physically and emotionally for the unknown of what was involved in the clinical trial. This was a new and welcome experience as none of his local doctors used the Internet to communicate. Laura communicated whenever she thought of something that would make it easier for Harris prior to his arrival in Cleveland. Other e-mails that helped to prepare him were:

Subject: Updates
Date: Mon, 15 Feb 1999 06:48:02 -0500
From: Laura, RN@cc.ccf.org
To: RHarris@trock.com

Good morning! Hope your golf outing and Valentine's Day was fun. Tenacity is a wonderful thing to have! We'll have to find you someplace special to have your anniversary dinner. We'll work on that soon, so you can get reservations made (Friday night!).

I am sending you treatment info, and videos made by the pharmaceutical companies to view while you are at home. You'll get the airborne packet on Tuesday. If you watch them Tuesday evening, we can talk Wednesday afternoon.

3:15 or 3:30? Do you have that function on your phone at work, and is that possible for both you and Betty, your wife to conference with me? Just let me know. If not Wed, what about Thurs at 11:00, 3:00 , or 3:30? Have a good day!
Laura

PS. I need to get a pharmacy phone number so I can phone in prescriptions. Thanks!

Laura was empowered to create and develop a relationship with him that would enhance his compliance in the trial. Of course, he would do as he was told. After all, his options were severely limited at that time in his life. But he did not feel alone or insecure as he was preparing to leave everything familiar, pack up for a month, move to another city, live in a hotel and subject himself to biological therapy that had unpleasant side effects. The frequent communication with Laura opened a door and engaged him in such a way that he felt as if he were on a team and not alone and isolated.

Another e-mail Laura sent had the following helpful hints:

Subject: Fax etc.
Date: Tue, 16 Feb 1999 06:49:34 -0500
From: Laura, RN@cc.ccf.org
To: RHarris@trock.com

Good morning! Thanks for the pharmacy phone number, I phoned in several Rxs yesterday. You should have a fax waiting for you at your office. It has your appointment schedule. Let me know before noon if you haven't gotten it (page me). You should also get an airborne package today. I have also included a shopping list of "things to bring." Let me know if you have any other questions, I'll be out of the office from today at
12:00 until tomorrow at 12:00. Thanks!

Airborne: 1-800-247-2676
airbill # 00975428
(sent to your home address)

Rxs at Walgreens:
Ibuprofen 800 mg TID on Mon and Thurs
Kytril 1 mg for Mon and Thurs if needed
Compazine 10 mg prn for nausea

Shopping list:
Tylenol 325 mg (any form)
Some kind of warm-up jacket, or "zipper down the front" sweatshirt (to keep you warm when you are "chilling")

Groceries:
Let me know if you need directions to a grocery store here in Cleveland.
chicken soup broth or bouillon cubes
juice or other clear liquid
Dick, keeping up your liquids is very important (I tried to insert a smiley face, but couldn't find the right button!) crackers, pretzels, party mix or other salty munchy

I think that does it for now. Have a good day!!!!!
Laura

Harris arrived for his visit better prepared than he could ever have imagined. He had his schedule and felt in control of the situation. He realized he was delighted with the use of e-mail to communicate as it meant that he and Laura were able to communicate whenever it was convenient to their personal schedules. It was much more effective than trying to speak by phone when both have very hectic lives. He found no loss of personalization via the computer. Instead, he found himself asking her questions in e-mail that he may have not discussed on the phone due to shyness.

What Harris found the most valuable was the independence Laura brought to the relationship. She was empowered to take charge. When there was a problem, she owned the problem and could resolve it. Too many times in his previous health care relations, the clinical staff would not assert themselves much without always communicating the need to "check with the doctor." Although there are times that is appropriate, this relationship seemed much more interactive and powerful.

Case study: Midwest Clinic for Women

The Midwest Clinic for Women had experienced serious interpersonal conflict between members of the professional and support staff. A number of individuals were considered "hard to work with."

During an extended meeting with the full team, it was disclosed that midwives occupied a "no-persons" position. They were angry because the physicians did not treat them as fellow-professionals, plus support staff did not show them respect and provide the kind of assistance they felt they deserved and needed.

A discussion ensued concerning the role midwives play in the practice and the value they provide for meeting the range of preferences of different patients. Appropriate institutional support for their role was defined. As a consequence, the organization now has a better understanding for whom the midwives provide service, why they provide a specific range of services and how this range of services fit into a common practice that benefits patients and staff.

The ambiance of the practice has changed markedly. There is every reason to believe that this affected the experience of patients who received care.

One woman's experience

Empowering staff impacts everybody. In addition to any other efficiencies it adds to your practice, it can make a public relations difference to your patients, your public and your organization as a whole.

Consider the story of Ms. Natalie Watson, Vice President of Public Affairs at an investment company. She has a very busy schedule, traveling to Washington and New York every month. She volunteers at a women's resource center, mothers three children, and organizes her time to be able to provide support for her elderly parents.

Ms. Watson was aware that October is Breast Awareness Month. There are multiple national promotions encouraging women to schedule mammograms during this month, and marketing begins long before October. Women of all ages become aware of the need for mammograms as breast cancer screening through the use of print, television, radio, women's groups and billboards, just to identify a few vehicles.

Ms. Watson heeded the advice all around her. She called the hospital women's center to schedule her annual mammogram and was pleased they could accommodate her on the day of her choice. The appointment scheduler spent twenty minutes on the phone updating all information from the previous year. Ms. Watson was pleased that she could expedite her appointment by answering the questions and confirming her insurance information prior to her mammogram.

She also was pleased to be able to access the first appointment of the day, at eight a.m. As she said good-bye and was about to hang up the phone, the scheduler told her, "Please be here 20 minutes early the morning of your appointment." Ms. Watson asked, "Why do I have to be there 20 minutes before eight, that's so early?" The scheduler said, "We need to verify your information that day."

Ms. Watson said, " Didn't you just take all my information and input it into the computer? Why would I have to spend time providing it a second time?" She was told, "That's the way we do it, so please be there 20 minutes ahead of your appointment." Ms. Watson said, "You have taken up 20 minutes of my time. I'm not going to come in early. I will arrive immediately before my appointment."

According to Ms. Watson, the interaction disturbed her. It bothered her throughout the day. She felt as if she had been in an offensive conversation, even antagonistic in nature. All because she wanted to schedule a mammogram. And this was an exam that she would pay for; it was not complimentary. Somehow, the fact that it upset her made the whole episode even more annoying and memorable.

The day before her exam, she received a phone call. "Ms. Watson, this is the women's center, would you please give us a call? This concerns your mammogram appointment." She called back and was told that somehow she had been dropped from the computer appointment list, and she was no longer scheduled for first thing in the morning. She was asked if she would mind rescheduling two hours later. She politely told them that she had planned for the eight a.m. appointment and had other plans for later in the day. She was then asked what other day she would like to come in for her exam. She told them, "I am not a very happy camper. I booked this two weeks ago, planned for it and now the day before, you're telling me my time slot is not available?" The staff person said, "Yes that's right. We are sorry, but that's what happened. Now when would you like to reschedule?"

Ms. Watson said, "When is the next available appointment?" Fortunately, it was in two days time and she was available. However the appointment person then said, "I have some questions to ask you to make sure we have all of your current information." Ms. Watson said, "I provided that information when I scheduled my original appointment. I don't have time to spend on the phone doing it again." The scheduler then said, "Please be here 20 minutes before your appointment."

By this time, Ms. Watson was very frustrated. "Why should I have to go in early to supply information I've already provided?" she wondered. "I've spent too much of my time trying to schedule this appointment—20 minutes on the phone scheduling the original appointment, plus another 20 minutes on the phone today. Now they are asking me to come in 20 minutes early to provide the same information."

"This makes no sense," she told the appointment scheduler. To which the scheduler replied, "A lot of people tell me the same thing. I think it's foolish too. But you need to tell somebody who can do something about it. I'm just doing what I'm told is my job."

Ms. Watson told at least ten people how frustrated she was trying to make an appointment to get a mammogram at this particular women's center. "You know," she said, "there are many places in our community where I can get a mammogram. I have gone to this facility because I believe their radiologists are well trained. And it is my understanding that their mammogram center is credentialed and has high-quality equipment. I want to give myself every opportunity when I take the time to have a mammogram. I want to limit as many opportunities for errors as possible. But they certainly aren't focused on the needs of the corporate woman or anyone with a busy schedule.

"On top of that, the person on the phone was not empowered to do anything about the situation. In the future, I'm going to research where else I might have my mammogram with equally credentialed staff and a greater sensitivity to the needs of the patient."

When Ms. Watson went to her appointment, the technician apologized for not having her previous films available. The technician told Ms. Watson, "It's too bad you had to cancel your appointment the other day. We had your films that day, but they were sent back to the warehouse when you didn't show up."

Ms. Watson said, "But it was the women's center that canceled my appointment. Does this mean that my mammogram cannot be interpreted?" "Oh no," the technician said, "but the doctor will want to wait until we can get your old films so she can compare them from last year to this year. It will take an extra day or two, but it is better for you. Because you had an unpleasant experience at our facility, I will ask Dr. Blue to call you personally with her findings. She won't mind doing that, and I think it'll set your mind at ease. Please accept my apologies on behalf of our radiology department for the trouble you had arranging your appointment. I will take on the responsibility of writing this up, sending it to our administrator and seeing if we can give our appointment system some serious attention. Thank you for sharing the details of your experience. Again, I regret that we didn't do a good job."

Ms. Watson left with very mixed feelings. She really wanted her mammograms done at this facility. She had confidence in the radiologists. She was pleased that the technician cared about how she was affected by her experience. But she is uncertain whether she will return to this center for her mammogram. After all, why should she go through the hassle of dealing with an appointment staff who isn't empowered to make a difference?

This is clearly a problem for the radiologist who was held responsible for the system when in reality, the system is run by the hospital. Yet in the eyes of the patient, they are one and the same. If the hospital employee had been empowered to own and fix the problem, one woman could have had a very different experience.

Chapter 6

The Three Rs—Retreat, Research, Reorganize

"If you don't know where you're going, you'll probably end up somewhere else."
— Yogi Berra

Strategic planning retreat

In business, as in war and politics, strategy is the term used for a comprehensive plan of action that will lead to long-term success. In the same vein, strategic planning is one of the most vital steps to marketing your practice.

As we enter the new millennium, many group practice managers realize they can no longer afford a "business as usual" mentality. Faced with declining revenues, increasing competition and consolidations due to merger activity, they're working closely with their physician boards and managers to determine how to maintain net income, while still growing the practice and competing for managed care contracts and patients.

Holding a retreat is one important first step in the strategic planning process. The goal of such a retreat, obviously, is to make sure all of the physicians are reading from the same page. In addition, a retreat allows you to: identify the current status of the practice, along with opportunities for improvement; develop consensus on where the practice wants to be in the future; get group agreement to design an action plan; and make a commitment to dedicate the resources to implement it. A strategic retreat also can help your group develop customer insight, competitor intelligence and broad environmental assessments.

There may be times when a retreat is used for very basic and tangible issues which are impacting the practice. These may include such concerns as: the ultimate size of the group; the geographic area it wants to serve; its relationship with the hospital; physician compensation models; and marketing strategy.

Often, even small steps can be very powerful. A practice may decide that the most important thing it can do is form an executive committee to streamline decision-making. Or it may focus on ways to bring non-medical staff into the decision-making process. Whatever important issues the practice faces may be an appropriate subject of a strategic retreat.

A retreat involves a creative problem-solving process. It allows you to identify options and to make choices. It allows you to select specific opportunities, generate ideas and create a plan of action.

As your group works to identify issues and goals during a retreat, everyone must participate in the "brainstorming." There are a few rules that apply to this process. Deanna Roberts, president of Roberts Communication Group, Tampa, FL, and a leader in corporate consulting, uses examples to create a visual picture. She shares the following insights.

Most people have to be led through a process that looks like this if you want them to become long-term customers or partners.

1. Awareness: Cut through the clutter to present a simple message.

2. Interest: Created when the partner sees his/her stake in the message being created.

3. Knowledge: If the partner has gone through the previous two phases, now he/she is willing to learn more.

4. Caring: The act of buying a product or service does not necessarily create a long-term relationship with the seller. The goal is to capture people emotionally as well as intellectually, to make them see they are part of an important vision and mission and to convince them to act in support of that mission.

5. Involvement: When people choose to be involved, they put a part of themselves into an organization. The key is to find everyone's level for involvement and invite them to participate.

6. Commitment: You can expect an ongoing, sustainable relationship. A committed partner is one who will remain when short-term benefits are not readily apparent, or worse, when the organization is under attack. That is partner loyalty. Long-term commitment and loyalty are earned through a multilevel, continuous process.

"It's a tried and true maxim that people support what they create."
— Margaret J. Wheatley, chaos theorist

To provide the most comprehensive information about strategic retreats, I've asked my colleague, Barbara Ann Blue, to contribute her extensive expertise to this chapter.   She is an attorney who founded and now serves as president of Business Performance Group, Inc., a management and organizational consulting firm. Ms. Blue's company specializes in improving organizational effectiveness and in leading organizations through change. It also develops high-performing leaders and teams, creates better outcomes by facilitating group consensus, and promotes problem-solving and conflict resolution.

Possible future mailer.

"The only constant is change"

How do you know when it's time to think strategically about the future of your group practice? Here are some key indicators to help you decide if the time is right:

- You're working harder and making less money than you used to.
- Your colleagues are opting for early retirement or changing careers or considering career alternatives. (Haven't you always wanted to run a bookstore?)
- You are losing patients.
- You are not getting your share of new patients in the marketplace.
- You're spending more time on paperwork than patient care—or at least it seems that way.
- You are experiencing high turnover in staff and spending more and more time on recruiting, training and re-training.
- You are thinking about reorganizing your practice.
- It isn't any fun anymore.

The fact that the world is changing comes as no surprise. The speed at which it is changing is what is mind-boggling. This is evidenced by the fact that what you did last year doesn't seem to work anymore. When there is a business imperative that is pushing you to think, "We have to do some things differently or we won't be here five years from now," it's definitely time to reflect on your future.

So what do you do? How can you reflect when your work is consuming so much of your time?

What about getting away from your practice—with others—and spending time considering how to position your practice to develop and sustain a competitive advantage in spite of the never-ending change? Think you can't afford the time and expense? I suggest that you can't afford not to invest if you want to be in business in five to ten years. The best option is to set aside at least a day or two for strategic thinking and planning, followed by at least quarterly updates to see how you are doing.

What benefits can you expect from your efforts to plan strategically for the future? You will have the:

- Chance to examine what's been working well and what has not.
- Opportunity to gain insights from your customers (patients, staff, referring physicians, hospital administrators, managed care companies, the doctors in your group).
- Opportunity to identify emerging trends and marketplace needs and decide which of these your group is best suited to take advantage of now and in the future.
- Chance to openly talk about the threats to your ongoing success and what you need to do to meet the seemingly ever-growing challenges.
- Chance to bring your group into clear alignment around what your purpose should be, what you want to create together for the future, the kind of values you want to integrate into all parts of your operation, and the three to five key strategies on which your group needs to focus its energy and resources in order to make the biggest difference.

In other words, everyone associated with your group will be on the same page—working toward the same goals and the same future. It also will enable you to establish clear accountabilities and time frames. The old adage that "people support what they create" is true. Given a clear direction and the opportunity to see where they can contribute, people in an organization usually will pull together to make it happen.

Preparing for the strategic planning retreat

Once you've decided to schedule a strategic planning retreat, the following steps should help you avoid pitfalls and help you achieve the outcomes you want.

Decide who should be there.

When thinking about who should be involved, I recommend that you err on the side of inclusiveness without getting so large that the size makes serious conversation and strategic thinking unwieldy. Consider whose thinking you would want to help forge your group's future. Also think about who will be significantly impacted by changes in the way you operate and do business. If someone could significantly dampen your possibilities of success if he/she didn't get on board and support the changes, it's a good chance that person should be a part of the strategic planning process.

Survey your customers in advance.

You may need to spend some time thinking about who your customers really are since the changing industry brings new players to the table. Knowing what key customers think about your practice and the future of health care before the retreat can help guide your thinking during the retreat.

Review current literature related to your practice or emerging trends in health care.

So much is happening in health care, it's hard to stay on top of it all. Nevertheless, it is important to know what is happening and where the health care profession seems to be heading. If you can't do it all yourself, ask others to help and divide up professional magazines, news magazines, an Internet search and other sources that may speculate about the future of health care in the United States. Then, prior to the retreat, circulate the best as pre-reading to help stimulate thinking.

Identify a place.

Pick a place which is away from the hub-bub and which will be conducive to reflective thought. The location needs to be away from phones, televisions and pagers. I know that may seem impossible but, in reality, no one is irreplaceable for two days. So do whatever it takes to get your practice covered by others so you and other retreat participants will be disturbed only in a true emergency that no one else can handle.

Determine the length of time.

As I mentioned before, plan at least one or two days, preferably two. Reflective thinking is enhanced if enough time is allowed for thorough discussion of complete ideas and group consensus on decisions. Consider beginning on a Friday afternoon, carrying on into the evening and continuing on Saturday. Recognize going in that strategic planning is a journey, not an event, and you may need more than one session. If so, plan the sessions close together, so you don't lose momentum.

Consider hiring an outside facilitator who is a process expert with strategic planning experience.

This enables everyone attending the retreat to stay focused and participate in re-thinking the group's practice to meet changing demands and expectations. The facilitator should:

- Help the retreat planner(s) identify the outcomes hoped for as a result of the strategic planning retreat as well as who should attend;
- Advise the retreat planner of room arrangements and equipment needs;
- Learn as much as possible about your practice before the retreat;
- Help you identify perceived trends that are likely to impact your operation;
- Conduct confidential interviews with all retreat participants to gain their insights into the practice as it exists now and where they see the challenges and opportunities for the future; and
- Conduct similar confidential interviews with other key stakeholders such as patients, affiliated hospitals, referral sources, other employees, etc.

Ask internal interview questions.

Figure 6-a

Medical Specialty Partners interview questions

The following is a sample of the interview questions that might be used by a mythical practice called Medical Specialty Partners. Use this to compose your own interview questions.

1. What attracted you to Medical Specialty Partners?

2. What do you like best about working at Medical Specialty Partners?

3. What do you like least?

4. If you could work in an "ideal" work environment, what values would permeate the organization to make it such a special place for you?

5. An organization's mission is its reason for being—its purpose or why it exists. From your perspective, how would you describe the mission of Medical Specialty Partners?

6. To fulfill the mission you just described, what do you see as the major challenges/obstacles facing Medical Specialty Partners?

7. Looking 10 years out: If Medical Specialty Partners was an unpara leled success—the best company of its type in the world—what would that look like? What would be happening?

8. Looking at the CEO, as the leader of the company and this team, what do you see as his/her greatest strengths?

9. What suggestions would you offer the CEO that you believe would help him/her be an even more effective leader than he/she is now?

10. For you to consider the upcoming retreat to be time very well spent, what outcomes would you hope we could achieve together?

Analyze the information from all the interviews to identify key themes or trends.

Sharing this information at the beginning of the retreat helps participants see what they share in common and then build on these shared views, rather than on differences.

Set goals for the retreat.

Once the analysis is complete, determine the goals for the retreat and the process that will best help your workshop participants meet these goals in the t me available.

Create the initial design for the retreat.

Review the interview trends or themes and the initial retreat design with you or whoever is leading the group's strategic planning efforts. Make whatever changes are agreed upon as a result of this discussion and finalize the retreat design.

Send out appropriate pre-reading to help prepare participants for the kind of thinking that will be needed in the strategic planning effort.

This might include articles on the value of developing a shared vision of the future, trends affecting health care, how to stay competitive in a changing wor d—anything that might help to make the time together in the workshop more meaningful and productive.

Prepare appropriate materials to help participants stay on task.

Facilitate the retreat.

Debrief with the retreat planners and suggest where to go from there and a path to follow.

Content of the retreat

"A simple definition of a learning organization is a group of people continually enhancing their ability to create what they want to create."

— Peter Senge, author, *The Fifth Discipline*

Typically, the goals of the strategic planning retreat include: the alignment of the participants around the purpose of the practice (their mission); what they want to create together for the future (their vision); and the key strategies on which the group should focus to fulfill the mission and achieve the vision (strategic goals). Together, these make up the core values the group will embrace to help guide how they work together and with others as they fulfill their mission and pursue their vision and key strategies.

The retreat agenda might look like this:

- Stage-setting comments by the group's leader(s) and the facilitator;
- Review of goals and the agenda;
- Creation of ground rules to help participants work together effectively;
- Review of the interview data—themes/trends;
- Development of consensus around the mission of the practice—why it exists or should exist;
- Alignment around a vision for the future of the practice, which usually includes the creation of a vision statement;
- Consensus on the core values or guiding principles that will guide all employees of the practice as they work together to fulfill the mission and vision;
- Identification of the key strategic goals that need to be accomplished within three years to keep the practice on track and focused on what is most critical to its short- and long-term success; and
- Assignment of accountability for accomplishing each goal.

Let's look at these one by one.

Mission

The creation of a mission statement helps everyone understand why your group practice exists. The conversation around the development of the mission statement is sometimes as important as the mission statement itself. Your "reason for being" five years ago may not be the same as your reason today.

To review what has already been discussed in Chapter 4, your mission statement should describe why the organization exists (its core purpose), what service(s) and/or product(s) it offers, and to whom the service(s) and/or product(s) are offered.

Your mission may also specify by whom the service(s) and/or product(s) are offered, how its accomplishments are to be measured and in what geographic area the service(s) and/or product(s) are offered. The mission serves as the pivot point upon which all the objectives and strategies are balanced.

A good mission statement should meet most, if not all, of the following criteria:

- The mission statement is clear and understandable to all stakeholders (hospitals, patients, referring physicians).
- The mission statement, typically, is brief enough for most stakeholders to keep in mind.
- The mission statement clearly specifies why your group practice exists.
- The mission statement reflects your group practice's distinctive competence.
- The mission statement is broad enough to allow flexibility in implementation but not so broad as to permit a lack of focus.
- The mission statement serves as a template and the means by which your organization's leaders and stakeholders can make decisions.
- The mission statement is consistent with the values, beliefs and philosophy of your organization and the stakeholders.
- The mission statement engages each employee's personal commitment.

See Figure 6-b, for examples of mission statements from other organizations, some health-related, some not.

Figure 6-b
Mission statement samples

AARP (American Association of Retired Persons)

AARP is a nonprofit membership organization of persons 50 and older dedicated to addressing their needs and interests. We seek through education, advocacy and service to enhance the quality of life for all by promoting independence, dignity and purpose.

American Heart Association

The mission of the American Heart Association is to reduce disability and death from cardiovascular diseases and stroke.

AT&T

We are dedicated to being the world's best at bringing people together- giving them easy access to each other and to the information and services they want and need — anytime, anywhere.

Bay Health Systems

The mission of Bay Health Systems is to provide comprehensive services which maintain and improve the physical and mental health of all people who come to us in need.

Dermatology Partners, Inc.

We affiliate with premier dermatology practices to share innovative, value-added business and clinical expertise, in order to position them as providers of choice and centers of excellence for comprehensive medical, surgical and cosmetic skin care.

Gerber

The people and resources of the Gerber Products Company are dedicated to assuring that the company is the world leader in, and advocate for, infant nutrition, care and development.

Group Health Cooperative of Puget Sound

Group Health Cooperative is a consumer-governed organization whose mission is to enhance the well-being of patients and other customers by providing quality, cost-effective, pre-paid health care.

Intermountain Health Care, Inc.

Excellence in the provision of health care services to communities in the Intermountain region.

Merck

We are in the business of preserving and improving life.

Wal-Mart

We exist to provide value to our customers and to make their lives better via lower prices and greater selection; all else is secondary.

Washington Gas

To Provide the Best Energy Value - a superior product and quality service at a competitive price.

Vision

As noted before, a vision statement is a declaration of a desired future state of the organization—the future you want to create. It is based on reasonable beliefs as to what is worthwhile, challenging and inspirational. In *Built To Last,* the authors, Collins and Porras, say the following about vision:

"When properly conceived, vision is broad, fundamental and enduring; a good vision should serve to guide and inspire the organization for years.. A vision is a perpetual guiding star; not to be confused with specific goals or business strategies. The primary role of vision is to guide and inspire."

For your practice an effective vision should:
  • Be compelling;
  • Engage your hearts and your spirits;
  • Assert what you and your colleagues want to create;
  • Represent something worth going after;
  • Provide meaning to the work that people associated with the group/practice do; and
  • Be simple.

Figure 6-c includes examples of vision statements created by a variety of organizations.

Figure 6-c

Vision statement examples

Avon

To be the Company that best understands and satisfies the product, service and self-fulfillment needs of women globally.

British Airways

To become the world's favorite airline.

Dermatology Partners, Inc.

We will create the model for excellence in dermatology.

Group Health Cooperative of Puget Sound

By the year 2000, Group Health Cooperative will be the nation's best managed health care organization. We will have the most-satisfied customers. Our customer governance structure will be a national model for the collaborative delivery of cost-effective, quality health care. We will be the Northwest's most-desirable health care system in which to work. We will deliver and be recognized nationally for delivering quality health care to all segments of our population.

Inova Health Systems

To develop a comprehensive integrated health care system that will provide services superior to those available from any other source.

Intermedia Communications, Inc.

Working together to reinvent communications, advance understanding and shrink the world.

Lowes (Subsidiary of Alex Lee, Inc.)

To run our stores so well that customers make Lowes' Foods their primary place to shop.

Mayo Foundation

Mayo aspires to provide the best medical care through practice, education and research, in a unified, multi-campus systems.

Westin Hotels & Resorts North America

Year after year, Westin and its people will be regarded as the best and most sought after hotel and resort management group in North America.

Core values

> *"Good thoughts are no better than good dreams, unless they can be executed."*
>
> — Ralph Waldo Emerson

Core values define how the people associated with your practice "behave" in their dealings with others. They describe how people relate with others inside the organization and outside the organization. Core values are easily understood statements which:

- Describe how the group practice will behave while accomplishing its mission and vision;
- Set standards of excellence;

- Reflect high ideals;
- Are ambitious;
- Inspire enthusiasm; and
- Encourage commitment.

When thinking about core values, it sometimes helps to ask yourself: Which of these values would we aspire to for a hundred years, regardless of changes in the external environment or even if the environment ceased to reward us for having these values, or perhaps even penalized us? Conversely, which values would we be willing to change or discard if the environment no longer favored them? These questions can help you identify which values are authentically core. When articulating core values, the key is to capture what is authentically believed, not what other organizations set as their values or what the outside world thinks the values should be.

Core values are fundamental, intrinsic and help clarify the culture of the organization and what it truly values. To create an authentic set of core values is difficult. To live them on a day-to-day basis and have them permeate your organization is an extraordinary, but worthwhile, challenge. To make that happen, core values have to be more than words on a piece of paper. Conversations need to be held frequently to check to see how you are doing. Practices should ask their stakeholders regularly: "To live these values fully, what do we need to start doing, stop doing or do more of?"

At internal meetings, one or more of the values should be raised each t me you gather in order to raise the level of importance and check to see how you are doing. Core values should be used to help recruit, hire and orient new employees. They also should be incorporated into performance development processes, and included in training, promotion, compensation and succession planning decisions. In other words, they should truly be "core" to how you operate your practice. Creating core values is not a process to be taken lightly. Figure 6-d provides some samples.

Figure 6-d

Core values samples

Support and encourage my network of partners

Business Performance Group

- We exceed our customers' expectations—every time.
- We continuously learn and improve—treating success and failure as opportunities for growth.
- We live in integrity—practicing what we preach, as individuals and as a company.
- We communicate openly and constructively—valuing differences and resolving conflicts for mutual gain.
- We balance our lives—blending professional, personal, family and community goals.
- We each own our individual results and the company's results.
- We support each other—professionally and personally.
- We profit from this enterprise—financially and personally.
- We count our blessing and celebrate our successes.
- We have fun.

Dermatology Partners, Inc.

We are:
- Committed to excellence and dedicated to service.
- Guided by honesty and integrity.
- Dependent on teamwork and open communication.
- Dedicated to treating people with respect and dignity.
- Focused on building long-term relationships.
- Oriented toward growth through creativity and innovation.
- Relentless in the pursuit of our mission.

Group Health Cooperative of Puget Sound

In support of our mission, we believe in:
- A partnership of consumers, medical staff and employees committed to quality in all aspects of our endeavors.
- Providing services that are professional, caring, efficient and appropriate for all our patients and other customers.
- Meeting the needs of our patients and other customers, constantly trying to ensure their satisfaction and well-being.

- Maintaining a diverse work force in an environment that is safe, rewarding and stimulating.
- The right and responsibility of individuals to participate in decisions affecting their own health.
- Health promotion, education and prevention as key elements in our services.

Minnesota Consolidated Health Care

- We respect diversity and the value of each individual.
- How we achieve results is as important as the results themselves.
- We take personal responsibility for our actions and pride in making a difference.
- We work together as a team committed to open, candid communication and mutual support.
- Our successes are measured by our ability to exceed internal and external customer expectations.
- We act with honesty and integrity.
- We protect the environment and improve the quality of life where we work and live.

Sentara Health System

SERVICE: We are committed to help the sick and needy by providing superior service to our patients and our community with skill, concern and compassion.

QUALITY: Because our patients are our primary concern, we will strive to achieve excellence in everything we do.

PEOPLE: The men and women who work as employees, volunteers, physicians and students are the source of our strength. They create our success and determine our reputation. We will treat all of them with respect, dignity and courtesy. We will endeavor to create an environment in which all of us can work and learn together.

STEWARDSHIP: Fulfilling our mission requires that we use our resources wisely and with accountability to our publics.

INTEGRITY: We will be honest and fair in our relationships with all those who are associated with us, and other health care providers as well.

Strategic goals

Once a group has developed consensus around its mission, vision and values, it should turn its focus toward establishing priorities for how to achieve its goals. Thinking long-term about what the organization needs to accomplish leads to the creation of specific goals on which to focus energy and resources.

Strategic goals need to be specific enough to be measured and to represent an end result you plan to achieve within three years. Strategic goals answer the questions:
- What and where does the organization want to be in three years?
- What are the most critical areas on which we should focus our energy and resources in order to fulfill our mission and achieve our vision?

Retreat follow-up

Remember, strategic planning is a journey, not an event. Therefore, the process doesn't end with the retreat. In fact, in many ways it is just beginning because the only real value in developing a clear alignment around mission, vision, values and goals is what you do with it when you leave. You have created the framework for the plan and for the culture of your practice. Now it's time to put the meat on the bones and make it come alive.

Depending on the size of the practice and level of detail needed to ensure implementation, there may be one more planning step—identifying the specific steps needed (including who needs to do them and in what time frame) to make each tactical objective happen. This step is typically needed in larger practices where multiple people will be responsible for the accomplishment of various tactical objectives. It helps clarify responsibilities, time frames, and when different people or parts of the practice need to work together to move the practice toward its goals.

Making the plan come alive

"Skate to where the puck is going to be, not where it's been."
— Wayne Gretzky

How do you make the mission, vision, values and supporting plan come alive and stay alive? The final challenge comes in ensuring that the mission, vision, core values and key strategies actually drive the practice and its decisions.

That means they have to be discussed frequently to check to see how you are doing. Do the decisions you are making support your mission, move you toward your vision, reflect your core values, and help you achieve your strategic goals? Have you incorporated your core values into your recruiting, selection and orientation of new employees? Have you built your core values into your employee performance development, training and compensation programs? Are you accomplishing your objectives in a timely way? Are your mission, vision and core values part of everyday conversation?

If the answer to these questions is "yes," you are well on the way. If they aren't, dust off the strategic plan and get started before the competition leaves you in the dust.

If your plan has been well thought out, at least 80 percent of what the practice does should be directly connected to your mission, vision, core values and strategic goals. If that is the case, you will be well on your way to creating a sustainable competitive advantage for your practice and its stakeholders.

Case Study: A tale of two hospitals

A few years ago, two hospitals in a large metropolitan community merged. For purposes of this story, we will call these hospitals Carlton and Monroe. The CEO of the new entity (we'll call him Jim Thompson) was the CEO of Carlton Hospital before it merged with Monroe. Both hospitals had between 500 and 600 beds and had been owned by a larger out-of-state entity.

Jim called us to see if we could help move the two hospitals through the turmoil as quickly as possible with minimal disruptions. In addition to speed, he recognized the anxiety of management and employees at both hospitals. He wanted to institute a change process that valued the input of existing employees while creating an institution that could stay competitive in an increasingly competitive health care industry.

As is the case with many mergers, some of the cost efficiencies would come from the reduction in the number of top managers. The new entity clearly didn't need two CFOs, Vice Presidents of Human Resources, or Directors of Patient Care (to name just a few of the roles considered duplicative). The new entity did need the best leadership available and a clear direction for the future that everyone could rally around.

The first thing we did was to interview the CEO and members of the leadership team from both hospitals to: get a sense of their hopes and fears;

identify strengths and weaknesses of both entities; and determine threats to success and opportunities for creating and sustaining a highly competitive organization.

Then, we set aside two days for both leadership teams to retreat and think about where they needed to go in the future (vision), how they wanted to get there (goals) and the ideal structure to support the combined organization.

The CEO set the stage by assuring everyone that he would work with them to create a good opportunity for them, either inside the organization or outside. The focus was on what it would take to create a "win" for the organization and all members of the leadership team, even if their job changed or went away.

We helped the group establish ground rules for the retreat to guide their behavior and to help them accomplish the desired outcomes of the retreat. The goals or desired outcomes were significant and meant the participants had to stay on task and focused on the good of the organization, not themselves. They agreed to:
- Come together as a team;
- Get to know each other better;
- Re-focus on who we are, where we're going and what we value; and
- Commit to planning.

After sharing the interview trends that emerged from the confidential interviews conducted before the retreat, the next area of focus was on the existing corporate values. How important are they? Are our operations in sync with these values or not? And, what if anything is missing for this team as it moves forward?

Healthy conversation ensued around the existing values which were to: demonstrate respect; foster integrity; embrace change; enhance value; and lead through partnership. The discussion also helped to set parameters of what were important behaviors to make these values live through the scary process of consolidation.

The team agreed in advance that they would not finalize a vision statement but would identify common elements of a desired future that could be taken to all employees for consideration. The belief was that anyone who had a stake in this future ought to have the opportunity for input.

The leadership team envisioned the future by asking and answering:
- What are patients saying about us?
- Physicians are more committed and loyal than ever before. Why is that true?
- What are people saying about our physicians?
- We have succeeded in gaining a competitive advantage. What is it?
- Our employees have never been happier. Why is that?
- Our competitors feel threatened by our success. What are they saying about us?
- What does "corporate" say about us?
- How are we perceived in the community at large?

The leadership group came to consensus on the key elements that must be part of the consolidated hospital's future and then moved on to strategic goals to help achieve the vision. They answered the question: What strategic goals should we adopt for our consolidation efforts over the next two years? In doing so, they identified those areas of focus that would help them make significant progress in closing the gap between where they were, and where they wanted to be.

A cardinal rule of organizational development is that structure follows strategy. If an organization doesn't know where it's going, any structure will either get them there or not, depending on the people. So, once the vision, values and strategic goals were agreed upon, the team focused its attention on the organizational design needed to support the strategic direction. They started by generating as many ideas as possible to increase efficiencies and service levels through the new organization design. Then, in small groups, they were asked to design the ideal organization as if:
- This was their business (their patients, their physicians, their profits and losses, their reputations, and their credibility); and
- They were in it for the long-haul.

After the groups shared their thinking, everyone discussed the ideas that emerged and came together around criteria for evaluating options. They decided upon the following criteria for the organizational structure:
- Will it create or sustain competitive advantage?
- Will it move us closer to our vision?
- Will it improve quality and cost of patient care, physician relations, employee commitment, and community perception?
- Does it enable us to meet corporate's financial criteria?

Once the criteria was established, the leadership group evaluated the various design options and came to consensus around the organizational structure that made the most sense for them at that time.

To close, they agreed on the next steps needed for them to evaluate their own options and for communicating the thinking to the rest of the employees and gaining their input. The entire consolidation effort took less than three months.

Tactical objective acid test

Tactical objectives need to be specific enough to be measured and represent an end result you plan to achieve in one year. They should answer the question: what are the most important steps we need to take in the next year to move us toward the accomplishment of each strategic goal?

If you answer "no" to any of these questions, the tactical objective should be revised, deleted or moved to a later year:
- Does it relate to the MISSION?
- Is it IMPORTANT?
- Can it be ACCOMPLISHED IN 12 MONTHS?
- Will it attract COMMITMENT AND BUILD TEAM?
- Can we FUND it?
- Is it MEASURABLE?

Chapter 7

MARKET: Moving Forward—by Design
Working with Referring Physicians

"Your own words are the bricks and mortar of the dreams you want to realize."
—— Sonia Choquette

Obviously, you will have many different levels of relations with referring physicians. On the one hand, you may meet to discuss the formation of a network or a merger. Or, you may meet with someone else to negotiate relations as a preferred referral group. Each of these opportunities requires research, planning and a vision of what you want for your practice.

Once again, it is very important to stay in tune with the long-range plan for the practice. Ask yourself what outcome you want from the meeting. What do you have to do to position your group on a path to achieve your goal? What market research should you initiate prior to the meeting? You must know what you want for the group and how it applies to the long-range marketing plan.

Can certain behaviors move these referral relationships along? Definitely.

It sounds very basic. But remember, as noted before, referrals often are based on personal relationships. That being the case, it's important to be accessible and friendly to primary care physicians, whether in the medical staff lounge, at grand rounds, at committee meetings and at social outings. Also, look for opportunities to provide in-service presentations regarding a new technique or service to the staff of primary-care physicians in your community.

Consider the example of a successful orthopaedic group in Pittsburgh which did this very effectively. They developed dates when the athletic trainers employed by their group could visit with family practice clinicians to teach skills in bandaging, splinting and stretching. Together, the orthopaedists and the family practice physicians held a joint Saturday morning sports medicine clinic for their patients.   This same group of orthopaedic surgeons partnered with rheumatologists and the Arthritis Foundation to provide community lectures and support groups.   They found that building these relationships increased their referral base and kept it consistent.

It's also very important to track referring physicians.   Once you know who they are, you have a chance to acknowledge their referral patterns to you.   Studies show that referring physicians expect communication about the patients they send you, of course, but they also want to know you appreciate the referral.

Communicating also helps to maintain your group's professional relationships.   This is enhanced when you develop and implement a plan to keep in touch with referral physicians.   No matter how difficult it gets within a managed care system, referring physicians will always be a part of your patient care.   Obviously, it's in your best interest to nurture them carefully.   Here are some suggestions that will help you accomplish this:

- Spend time with referrers. Find out what's going on in their practices;
- Send brief periodic updates on how your group is adding locations, services, products or new physicians;
- Hold an open house for referral physicians' staffs;
- Partner with the hospital or a local university to conduct a CME program;
- Send letters introducing new practice associates and areas of the subspecialization they bring to your practice;
- Partner with a referring physician group to present informational talks at community groups;
- Volunteer for medical staff committees;
- Serve on community advisory boards and task boards relating to health in your community;
- Develop patient education materials in subjects that reflect the skill, knowledge and interest of your group and distribute them to health professionals;
- Be visible and available;
- Encourage every physician in your group to do one promotional activity a week, such as taking a referring physician to lunch or dinner; and
- Conduct a referral physicians' survey to find out if the referring physicians who send you patients are pleased with your services.

In addition to these ideas, there are other things you can do that will be of value to referring physicians.   For example, make it easy for referring physicians and their patients to use your services. If you joined a managed care panel after their booklet was printed, you have a perfect opportunity to write a personal letter and let your referrers know you are accessible and interested in their referrals. Let them know that you set aside a few time slots everyday for referred patients. Let your top referrers know that you understand that, when they need help, they need it now, not in two weeks.

At the same time, be sure to respect the referring physician's schedule. In addition to calling about a patient, you have other options. Information can be faxed or e-mailed. Both can be printed and added to the chart.

Whether or not you call a referring physician with your findings and recommendations, always send a prompt follow-up letter. And, one important thing I have learned from referring physicians after conducting numerous referral surveys: they appreciate an executive summary of your findings as you draft your report.

If you follow a patient for a long time, keep the referring physician informed about the patient's progress. If you find it necessary to refer the patient to another physician, let the primary practice know. Referring physicians find it annoying and upsetting to learn one of their patients has had surgery or hospitalization, and they have not been informed. It can be very embarrassing if the patient's family calls the primary doctor, and he/she has no idea what is taking place.

Referring physicians usually have spent years developing relationships with their patients. They know they'll be called to help the family sort through issues and complications. For that reason, if there's any way you can engage and partner with the referring physician in planning case management, always do it.

In addition to showing respect for the referring physician, find a way to say thank you for the continual interaction between your two practices. This can be done by writing a personal note of thanks, making an unexpected phone call to express your appreciation or by simply initiating a gesture that communicates your awareness of the relationship your practices share. Whenever possible and appropriate, praise the referring physician's alertness in picking up an abnormality. Be sensitive when talking to referred patients, as frequently what you say will be repeated back to the primary doctor. An off-hand remark or thoughtless statement may come back to haunt you.

Some specialists take the attitude that they're fixing a problem the primary care doctor can't solve. That certainly is not conducive to building positive referral relationships. Obviously, it is better for practice building if the specialist realizes this and instead, positions for a complementary relationship. Remember, everybody benefits when a referring relationship is open, honest and interactive.

To illustrate effective referral relationship marketing, I've called on the expertise of a long-time colleague, David Cassidy, Marketing Director for the Jewett Orthopaedic Clinic. A certified Athletic Trainer and a certified strength and conditioning specialist, Cassidy has worked as the strength and conditioning coach for the Orlando Magic along with being Medical Coordinator for the 1994 World Cup Soccer and 1996 Olympic Games (Orlando venue). He has served as Director of Operations for Sports Physical Therapy, Inc.(Florida division) and Manager of Marketing and Business Development for Orlando Regional Healthcare System. About seventy percent of Cassidy's role consists of helping his employers enhance relations with referral sources. Although his insight is offered primarily from the perspective of orthopaedics and rehab specialty care, I believe you will be able to translate it to your practice. The following discussion highlights some of his ideas.

Referral marketing example: Orthopaedics

The challenge for small- to mid-size orthopaedic practices is how to continue positioning the practice over time as an established practice and as a resource to your customers and community. One important factor you must understand is that your market strategies must reach further and have a greater impact than ever before and in multiple areas. In addition, you must be more creative with your time and talent than in years past.

Here are a few ideas that have been and continue to be successful in orthopaedic relationship marketing.

Physician-to-physician marketing

The old saying, "word of mouth is the best form of advertising," doesn't tell the whole story when discussing physician-to-physician based marketing strategies. Physician confidence and secondary referrals are based primarily on relationships. However, managed care has affected this dynamic as well, based on open or closed physician panels.

In Florida, many previously restrictive managed care plans have come full circle and no longer restrict specialty referrals. This change in policy reinforces the importance of strong physician-to-physician relationships to increase market share. Physicians who know one another and have rapport will use and refer patients to each other.

Nothing has a greater marketing impact or is a wiser use of time or dollars than an orthopaedic surgeon taking the time and effort to know his/her referring physicians. In fact, this referring customer is arguably your most important customer, next to your patients. This fundamental approach to marketing yourself and your practice will cost you valuable time but very little money.

Take, for example, a physician new to town who wants to establish a practice. The most productive marketing he/she can do is to acclimate to the new market and meet potential referring physicians. Whether entering a large practice or a solo office, this exercise produces dividends in patient referrals and creates a "connection" to other medical providers in the community. It takes the doctor out of the office for several half days when first starting office hours, of course, but most new physicians don't have a full appointment schedule, and their surgery schedule is usually light. Meeting face-to-face with another physician makes a tremendous difference and is extremely effective.

Another basic technique for marketing your practice is the "Thank you for the referral" note. This card or letter can be used as a tool to keep your practice on the top of the minds of referring physicians. The note, which can be on a simple note card, should be handwritten and offer a sincere expression of gratitude. Other effective correspondence should include pertinent clinical narratives which keep referring physicians informed of their patients' status.

Often, a conservative approach to care is initiated in the beginning, but after a certain amount of time or a special diagnostic test, the patient may need additional medical intervention or surgery. Because of the hectic pace in which physicians work, some fail to inform the primary referring physician of the next intervention into the patient's disease. Imagine how awkward it is for a primary care referring physician to discover that a shoulder or foot injury referred to a specialist six months ago has been surgically repaired, but he/she was not informed about it. Especially when the information comes from the patient, rather than the specialist's office!

To take this marketing opportunity one step further, as a surgeon, you can personally invite one or several of your referring physicians to join you in surgery as an observer. Although time usually prohibits the actualization of this invitation, the offer creates a tremendous impact. If by chance, the referring physician can clear a portion of the day to view the surgery, you will have forged a rock-solid relationship. In any case, whether you send a thank you note card or advanced clinical notes or share time in the operating room, referring physicians like to be informed and feel a part of the medical case management process.

Initiating other approaches to physician-to-physician marketing depends on your group's philosophy. There are several effective styles you can implement.

One style is the face-to-face approach, which can be very effective but labor intensive. The difficulty often is weighted on the side of the referral specialist. Obviously, it takes a great deal of time and effort to juggle the physician's schedule as well as his/her willingness to meet. For one thing, there are a number of other health care professionals, such as pharmaceutical reps, product vendors and surgical manufacturers, vying for the surgeon's time.

Often, the face-to-face interaction can be maximized over a scheduled lunch in the hospital or at a location selected by the referring physician. Another effective way to build the relationship is to bring lunch to the office of the referring physician where you can sit together and talk over lunch. This can be enhanced by also providing lunch for the office staff on the same day. It doesn't have to be a big deal. Simply bring pizzas or order deli sandwiches or trays. Before you go to this effort, be sure to ask the referring physician if it is okay and let the office manager know your plan in advance.

This soft approach to marketing can create a special relationship with the referring physician's practice and staff, which in turn can provide more expedient access to appointments for your patients. For a small- or medium-sized practice, creating access on the same day or the next day may be your competitive advantage over larger specialty practices.

Place yourself in the shoes of the referring physician who is positioned to refer his or her patient to a subspecialty practice. The physician has two choices: immediate medical referral or a non-urgent referral. An immediate referral would be a patient who presents to the primary care physician with an acute low back sprain/strain, torn ligament or cardiac work-up. In other words, this is a pathology that needs to be seen elsewhere quickly. The specialty practice that accommodates this type of patient and provides easy access to an appointment also makes the referring physician look good in the eyes of the patient and his/her family.

The non-emergency referral is the other choice. For that instance, you can provide referring physicians with collateral marketing materials in advance. These include prescription pads that include your office address(es), phone number(s) and location map(s). If possible, create them with duplicate backing so a copy remains in the primary care physician's files.

An updated managed care list also is very helpful to the referral physician's office staff. A referring physician who sends a patient to your office and your specific subspecialty only to discover the patient cannot be seen by your group because of managed care contracting will be upset and may cause you to lose a potential patient. Providing referral offices with a current list of the plans you are on eliminates this type of "oops" referral altogether.

In all these instances, your goal is to make the referral to your office as seamless as possible.

Physician-to-managed care marketing

Another marketing strategy that is worth reinforcing is building relationships with managed care companies. This process begins with constant monitoring of the demographics of the community. A managed care company with strong enrollment numbers may drop to a dangerous level, while a relatively new managed care company may move into the market as a result of an acquisition, thus becoming a major player in the market.

It is this type of market activity that should motivate your practice, as you sign up for managed care plans, to become a partner and develop collaborative relationships. It is more beneficial to be part of the process than simply on the panel. There are physicians and practices that have generated productive opportunities for themselves because of the effort they put into maintaining relationships with senior administrators and physician provider representatives.

For example, an executive with whom you have forged a good relationship may have a new opportunity with a managed care company. Once established, the executive may realize this managed care company does not have relations with your group. The executive then can create the conduit for your group to become more closely aligned with the managed care company.

Another example could occur when a capitation arrangement is awarded in your favor or the compensation cap rate is opened for discussion, based on the effort, energy and relationship your group has developed with plan administrators.

Physicians are often invited to participate in educational sessions or seminars concerning appropriate and non-appropriate referral patterns. This can result in a win/win experience for all parties. It is a bonus for the primary care physician to feel more confident and comfortable managing minor musculo-skeletal injuries. It is a win for the specialist who intervenes with the truly in-need patients.

Physicians and industry

A business opportunity that is frequently overlooked in many practices is the industrial medicine market. Mid-sized to large employers employ large numbers of employees who need a variety of services, such as pre-employment physicals, drug screenings, fitness assessments, ergonomic assessment of the work site and educational programs. Newer services being implemented are industrial and work site hygiene. Ergonomic assessment provides a wonderful opportunity to work closely with the company's safety director, risk manager and human resources director.

Your valued expertise can assist the company with its largest and most costly problem—lost workdays. As companies look for their competitive advantage, they also look for creative solutions. If the musculo-skeletal group can assist in the redesign of the workplace to create a safer and injury-free environment and reduce occupational injuries, a positive outcome is created. Also, employees receive the message that their employer cares about the health and safety of its work force.

The concept of working with referrers remains simple. You can and should spend time and resources developing other marketing initiatives. Yet, many of the more valued marketing efforts are started and nurtured by relationship marketing.

Figure 7-a

Sample Referring Physician Survey

FLORIDA **HEART** GROUP

1613 North Mills Avenue
Orlando, Florida 32803
407 894-4474
1-800-28-HEART (1-800-284-3278)

Referring Physician Survey

Dear Doctor:

Because we place great value on your referrals and your satisfaction with our service to your patients, we want to listen carefully to your thoughts and opinions. To help us serve you better, please take a few minutes to let us know your concerns, as well as those areas where you think we're doing a good job. A prepaid envelope is provided for you to return the survey to our marketing company for compilation. Thank you for your time.

1. When you recommend a cardiologist to a patient, how important are the following considerations? Please use the scale of 5 to 1 *with 5 being the most important.*

   a) Board Certification
      5   4   3   2   1

   b) Managed care panel participation
      5   4   3   2   1

   c) Personal knowledge of the specialist
      5   4   3   2   1

   d) Prompt feedback from the specialist
      5   4   3   2   1

   e) Facility/hospital privileges of the specialist
      5   4   3   2   1

   f) Timely return of the patient for follow-up care
      5   4   3   2   1

   g) Geographic location of the specialist
      5   4   3   2   1

2. Our records show that you have referred patients to the Florida Heart Group within the past 18 months.

   a) What was the primary reason you selected our practice?

      _____

      _____

   b) Were you satisfied with the level of service your patient(s) received?
      ___ Yes   ___ No

   c) Would you refer to our practice again?
      ___ Yes   ___ No

3. Please rate Florida Heart Group's service to you and your patients in the following areas, on a scale of 5 to 1 *with 5 being the highest.*

   a) Overall quality of care
      5   4   3   2   1

   b) Timely consults
      5   4   3   2   1

   c) Timely, written information on patient visit
      5   4   3   2   1

   d) Friendly, courteous staff
      5   4   3   2   1

   e) Timely appointment scheduling
      5   4   3   2   1

   f) Timely return of phone calls
      5   4   3   2   1

   g) Participation in the same managed care plan(s)
      5   4   3   2   1

   h) Patients referred back for follow-up care
      5   4   3   2   1

4. Which managed care plan has the highest volume of patients in your practice?

      _____

5. Are you aware that the Florida Heart Group has designed and built a new cardiac office building which provides outpatient cardiac services in an efficient setting for patients?
      ___ Yes   ___ No

(Continued on back)

Figure 7-a Cont'd

Sample Referring Physician Survey

6. Are you aware that the Florida Heart Group recently developed a Congestive Heart Failure Clinic, under the leadership of Mark Milunski, MD, to better serve the needs of your patients who have CHF?

    ___ Yes   ___ No

    a) Do you have patients who would benefit from this specialized service?

        ___ Yes   ___ No

    b) Do you think you would refer CHF patients to the Clinic in 1996?

        ___ Yes   ___ No

7. Do you feel a sense of cooperation by Florida Heart Group cardiologists as they work together to care for your patients?

    ___ Yes   ___ No

8. Please make any suggestions you may have concerning how Florida Heart Group can improve services to you, your staff or your patients.

    _____

    _____

    _____

    _____

    _____

    _____

    _____

    _____

    _____

    _____

    _____

    _____

    _____

Name _____
      (optional)

Phone _____
       (optional)

                                        Thank you.

Referral enhancement behaviors

Be respectful of the referrer. If you find something questionable about the patient's treatment, take it up privately with the referring physician. Unless it's medically necessary, don't repeat tests already performed, as this drives up costs and can be offensive to the referring physician as well as the patient.

Use basic marketing techniques. Print Rolodex cards and distribute them to your referring physicians to make it easy to reach your practice. Include your e-mail address and your fax number. Provide referrers with brochures which will be of value to their patients. Be sure to include a brochure rack to keep the referrer's office neat.

Monitor your referral patterns. Keep a log of who's referring and check it every month. If you discover that referrals from certain colleagues are declining, call to find out if you or your practice has in some way offended them.

Remember those who support your practice. It is not out of line to send a note or a gift certificate or to host referrers who have helped build your practice. You may send lunch to a referral physician's office, host a referrer's staff to a wine and cheese evening in your office or make a contribution in honor of physicians in your community.

Recognize that referred patients are ambassadors of your practice. When they return to the primary physician and are appreciative of the referral, it helps to build positive relations on your behalf. Create systems within your practice to see referred patients on time, treat them respectfully and communicate appropriately with referring physician.

Figure 7-b

Sample referral physician letter

(Note: This letter can be prepared by your transcriptionist from "key words" contained in the dictation. Deliver via fax and mail the original on the indicated date, along with a copy of the patient information brochure.)

(Date)

(Referring doctor name)
(Practice Name)
(Address)
(City/State/Zip)

RE: (Patient's Name)

Dear (Referring Doctor):

The above referenced patient was seen in our offices on (date of visit) presenting with symptoms, which indicate (diagnosis). S/he is being treated with (medication) and a course of surgical intervention is indicated.

I have recommended that (surgical procedure) be performed within (time period) and are staff is in the process of making the necessary preparations for (Mr./Mrs./Ms (patient's last name) surgery. Additionally, we will be scheduling a post – surgical visit(s) to evaluate the progress of this patient's recovery process.

Thank you for the confidence you have expressed in referring your patient to us. I will keep in touch with you re: (his/her) progress.

Sincerely yours,

(Name), MD
Vascular Surgeon

Case Study: Cardiology referrals

While working with a group of cardiologists in a community in the Midwest, the following scenario presented itself. A large primary care group practice was formally changing its relationship with a health system and developing its own network. Because of the size of the primary care group, each of the cardiology groups in town was positioning to re-establish its relationship and attempting to make it exclusive.

As the cardiology group prepared for a meeting with the CEO of the primary care group, they reviewed their referral relationship and realized the large financial impact they would suffer if they were replaced by another cardiology group.

A brainstorming session was conducted to develop strategies for the meeting. It included the cardiology administrator, the marketing director and the medical director. The meeting agenda included the following topics:
- Sharing perspectives on the current relationship;
- Identifying cardiology competitors and what values they could bring to a relationship with the primary care group;
- Defining who was to be empowered to be the decision-maker, in the eyes of the primary care group;
- Reviewing the current contract;
- Working the numbers to determine the impact of capitation versus fee-for-service;
- Overview of the primary care market demographics and its impact on cardiology;
- The game plan, goals and desired outcome for the meeting; and
- Focusing on the need to listen and ask questions about what primary care physicians want and need.

Both the administrator and the medical director of the primary care group attended the meeting. They expressed their concern about the community's awareness of their group once they became external and independent of the hospital. They discussed the roll-out of their marketing plan to educate the community about their newly developed identity and their availability to accept new patients. They were going to spend resources educating existing patients and encouraging them to remain with the primary care group. The plan was to position their primary care physicians with employers so that "If your employees don't have access to our group, you should go talk to your insurer."

This led to a discussion about how the primary care group would differentiate itself. They made a strong case for hoping to align with the specialty practices that had partnered with them previously. Although many specialty groups had initiated relations, the medical director's position was that he had loyalty to groups who served them well in the past and believed strongly that in a managed environment, no additional physicians were needed to serve the existing patient base.

The primary care group used the chaos in the marketplace to take a position of leadership. They believed that was how physicians retain their independence.

When the cardiology administrator asked the primary care administrator what he wished for, he responded:
- Rate relief;
- Loved the idea of mutual marketing;
- Open books, shared risk;
- Win-win-win;
- 80/20 rule—are we doing things right or could it be managed more efficiently; and
- Honesty and integrity.

After the meeting, it was recommended that the cardiology group should:
- Look at all the pieces of the puzzle;
- Evaluate the potential of the relationship, both financially and to collaboratively position as partners with the primary care group;
- Develop a list of differentiating qualities with value to the primary care group, patients, employers and insurers;
- Focus on the viability of capping cardiology care;
- Develop opportunities for mutual marketing;
- Maintain a weekly phone dialogue effort with the primary care group administrator and medical director; and
- Implement a game plan and timeline, as well as assign resources and tracking methods.

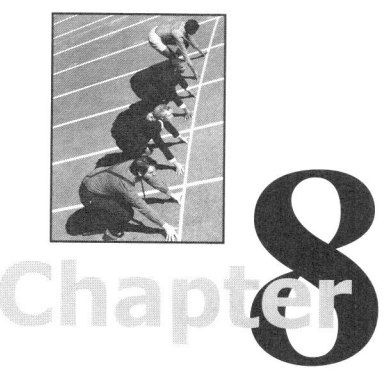

Chapter 8

Getting the Most from Your Relationship
with a Hospital or Health System

"Good things may come to those who wait, but only bad things left by those who hustle."

— Abraham Lincoln

Practices of every size and specialty can reap significant benefits by tapping into the resources available at most hospitals and health care systems. From technical support to marketing research to cooperative advertising, there are hundreds of marketing opportunities to benefit your practice.

Why should a hospital or health care system share its resources with your practice? Take a moment and consider this question before visiting your local hospital and requesting that they share their precious resources.

The answer is simple. There is strong competition for your business. Hospitals are well aware that physicians most often have a choice when it comes time to admit a patient to the hospital for inpatient and outpatient services. In today's managed care environment, almost every plan includes at least two hospital competitors per market region, sometimes more. If the physicians in your practice are competent and cost effective, there will always be more than one hospital seeking their business. That demand can be leveraged to benefit your practice.

However, it's important not to confuse leveraging the demand for your practice's business, with the concept of trading admissions for amenities. The former is acceptable. The latter is illegal. Physicians must decide which hospital to use based on what is best for the patient.

Because this chapter is dedicated to helping physicians and practice managers find and tap these marketing opportunities, I asked my colleague Bob Kodzis to share his insights, based on his role in marketing a hospital system.

Kodzis, with whom I have served on several health care marketing boards, is the founder of Flight of Ideas, a creative consortium dedicated to helping people and groups "break out of the box." The former Corporate Director of Marketing and Creative Services at Orlando Regional Healthcare System, he works with organizations and foundations across the U.S., providing them fresh, fun, creative ways to approach their challenges. In addition to his work with Flight of Ideas, he is a nationally recognized speaker and presenter. The following discussion summarizes some of his thoughts.

Building relationships

Hospitals and health care systems want your business. They want to build a long-term relationship with your practice (in spite of how it sometimes feels). They cannot buy your business. So they must be creative.

A number of hospital marketing directors have found very creative ways to strengthen relationships with members of their active medical staffs. Most do this by sharing information, knowledge and skills.

In a couple of unique and visionary organizations, marketing and business development managers have even developed sophisticated physician marketing service bureaus. These services are designed specifically to meet the marketing and information needs of loyal physicians. In the two examples that I have witnessed, both offered services and information to all physicians, but only actively promoted the opportunity to active admitting physicians.

In most cases, it will be up to the physician and the practice administrator to unlock the treasures available in most hospitals and health care systems. The key is to effectively leverage your practice's power.

The power of your practice is based on such factors as:

Relationships with hospital leadership

The stronger your relationship with the hospital leadership, the more likely you are to get what you need from the hospital. It's as simple and as logical as it sounds. Remember that the best long-term relationships are mutually beneficial. Spend some time assessing what benefits your practice has to offer.

Quality of medicine practiced

High-quality, cost-effective medicine is always a good way to get the attention of hospital leadership. You may need to clearly point out the strong points of your practice and your physicians, but once you do, you'll find hospital administrators more receptive. Hospitals will always seek strong relationships with strong practitioners. It makes them a more attractive package for managed care companies and large purchasers.

Reputation of physicians/practice

Never underestimate the power and the value of a good reputation. If your physicians are well known, well liked, well respected and or well published, your ability to negotiate is stronger. You can add positive exposure and good will by association to your stack of bargaining chips. I've seen practice administrators very effectively use this factor in negotiations: These are exactly the kind of physicians with which hospitals want to build a long-term relationship.

Annual hospital utilization

Physicians who admit a higher number of patients to a given hospital wield greater power than do their lesser admitting counterparts. It's only logical. They are better known by the hospital staff and leadership, and their business is valuable enough to protect and nurture. Use caution when leveraging this factor. The last thing you want is to appear to be tainting the clinical judgment and business loyalty of your practice.

Future/potential hospital utilization

This factor includes the growth potential of your practice, and the business that your practice currently sends to other hospitals. It is the least tangible of the factors, but it remains an important factor considered by hospital leadership when assessing the potential business value of a relationship with your practice.

Level of activity and visibility

The more visible and active your physicians are in the hospital environment and the community, the more likely the hospital leadership is to listen to your ideas and to engage in relationship-building dialogue. Being there is half the battle. Participating, constructively and visibly, is the other half.

Philanthropy

If your physicians and employees contribute a significant amount of time, talent or treasure in support of a hospital or a health system, your friends in the Foundation and volunteer offices will be more than happy to help you to get what you need.

Foundation managers are often excellent negotiators. Because of the amount of philanthropic revenue they are responsible for facilitating each year, Foundation leaders are powerful allies in the hospital environment. Volunteer offices do not have the financial power of the Foundation, but they can help navigate the system and find the right people.

All of these factors combined represent the cumulative negotiating power of your practice. Before attempting to unlock the treasures in your hospital or health care system, do a quick practice power inventory using these factors to guide you. Practices with strong negotiating stances (based on the previously noted factors) almost always will find it easier to share and benefit from hospital resources.

Although systems vary from market to market, four basic categories of treasure can be found at most hospitals and health care systems.

Information is power

All good marketing begins with good information. Hospitals and health care systems throughout the U.S. spend billions of dollars each year gathering, analyzing and reporting information that is critical to their success. Some of this information holds value for your practice. In most cases, the cost of sharing this information is very low and the benefit to the practice is high. The following are some of the many information treasures available in your local hospitals and health care systems:

- *Practice benchmarking*
  - If you knew that your physicians achieved the best outcomes in town and were among the most cost-effective practitioners in the country, how would you market your practice differently?
  - In most cases, best practices and benchmarking information are readily available to the physicians of your practice. You simply need to request it.
  - Most health systems conduct benchmarking studies designed to measure the performance of their hospitals and their physicians and to compare that performance against a national or regional standard. The ultimate goal of this process is to identify the best (most effective and cost-effective) practices and to encourage all admitting physicians to operate at a similar, high level of performance.
  - Most often, only a small amount of this information is regularly shared with admitting physicians. However, much of this information is readily available to any requesting physician. Individual results are confidential

and will be masked (with the exception of those pertaining to the requesting physician).

- Positive results can become good positioning tools for your marketing efforts. This information is relevant to referring physicians, medical networks, large employers and managed care providers.
- Negative results can be used to initiate a process improvement effort. Whether the results are negative or positive, it's important that you understand the measures being gathered on your physicians
- Where can you get this information? Departments most likely to have access to physician benchmarking information include: Medical Staff Services, Medical Staff Leadership, Strategic Value, Clinical Process Improvement, Quality Assurance.
- Caveat Marketer: Benchmarking is a very complex process. There is no guarantee that your hospital or health care system will employ the right methodology. Before you consider using this information to benefit your practice, be sure you know the source of the information, how it was processed and how it will be communicated.

- *Marketing research*
  - Marketing departments, marketing research departments and planning departments gather and archive an extraordinary amount of market intelligence. Professionals in these departments can tell you a great deal about the community, the business community, the medical community and the competitive environment. They can provide you with a load of good relevant market information including lists of top employers, top health concerns, the rate of community growth, areas of greatest community growth, etc.
  - The key to getting value from this information bank is to first understand what specific information you need to gather. What do you want and need to know? If you can articulate the parameters of the information that you'd like them to share, most marketing research professionals can custom-slice the data to meet your needs with very little effort.

- *Demographics*
  - Demographics are objective characteristics of a population. They include factors such as age, sex, race, income, education and size of household.
  - This information can be used to target specific age groups, ethnic groups and socioeconomic groups. While there are limits to the segmentation power of demographics, they continue to be a valuable tool as you

begin the process of segmenting your market and targeting only individuals and groups relevant to your practice.

- Most hospitals and health care systems use a great deal of demographic data. Some subscribe to annual demographic updates. As long as the information is not copyrighted, it will cost a hospital very little to provide your practice with reports and data. You simply need to find the keeper of the demographic data and ask.
- Where can you find this information? Demographics can be found most often in one of the following departments: Marketing Research, Marketing and Advertising, Management Information Systems, and sometimes Human Resources. (Demographics can be used for employee recruitment purposes too.)

- *Psychographics*
  - Psychographics is the art and the science of segmenting a population according to their lifestyles. Users of psychographic information argue that this form of segmentation is a far great predictor of buying behavior than traditional demographics.
  - There are a number of different psychographic models, but most divide a given population into 20-50 psychographic groups, or clusters. The names of the clusters are often illustrative of the group. They include colorful names, such as "Furs and Station-wagons," "Blue Bloods" and "Empty Nesters."
  - Information companies, including Inforum, The Sachs Group and National Research Corporation, market health care-specific psychographic information banks to hospitals. Typically, they target marketing research departments, marketing departments, managed care and administration.
  - These marketing information systems are packed with useful information on the entire market served by the health care system. Today most allow their clients access to even larger data banks using the Internet.
  - In addition to population and growth statistics, demographics and psychographics, these information companies provide hospitals with some rather sophisticated models to predict demand for specific health care services, market demand for physicians by specialty and even site assessments for facilities and practices.
  - This information, combined with these models and capabilities, can enhance the marketing efforts of almost any medical practice.

- It's always a good idea to request that the system programmer/operator print the parameters of the query in the headline of the report. This will assure that all readers understand how the study is defined.
- Where can you find this information? Not all hospitals use psychographic information. However, most large health care systems have at least one psychographic data system in-house. These lifestyle clusters and information can be found most often in one of the following departments: Marketing Research, Marketing and Advertising, and Management Information Systems.
- Caveat Marketer: A word of caution when using this information. The quality of the information is often dictated by the skill of the individual operating the system. Questions (called queries when posed to a computer) must be very carefully crafted to generate the focused and accurate market information you need.

- *Article clipping services*
  - Many hospitals hire media clipping companies to identify and archive articles, news stories and ads. Others have staff and volunteers clipping articles and setting VCRs to capture newscasts and competitive ads. Some hospitals keep their archives well organized and up-to date. Reviewing these archives on a regular basis will really benefit your frame of reference as you prepare to position your practice in the marketplace. Physician ads are often automatically clipped.
  - By gaining access to a hospital's clipping archives, you can stay abreast of what is current in the media and you can see how your competitors are positioning themselves in the marketplace. When you have the opportunity to look at six months worth of ad clippings, patterns and underlying strategies often become rather obvious.
  - Where can you find this information? Media clippings can usually be found in the Public Relations Department, Media Relations Department or in small hospitals, the Marketing Department or Administration. Advertising clippings can be found in the Public Relations Department, the Marketing Department or the Advertising Department.

Sharing skills and talents

- *Focus Groups*
  - Many hospitals conduct patient and community-based focus groups. These professionally facilitated group sessions help administrators and employees to better understand the perspectives of their customers and

community members. New concepts and advertising ideas are often tested in front of representative focus groups of actual and potential customers.

- If you enjoy a good relationship with a hospital that conducts regular focus groups, then you may have a unique opportunity to test ideas and witness, first hand, how the market responds to them. Some practices have learned to tap the power of this research tool well by working closely with hospital marketing researchers and focus group facilitators. I have facilitated many shared focus groups in which several clients contributed to, and benefited from the process.

- Who can you talk to about focus groups? Focus groups are most often conducted through the marketing, organizational development or marketing research departments of hospitals and health care systems. Sometimes outside consultants conduct focus groups in support of a project or initiative. I've found consultants to be less receptive to the concept of sharing their group processes, but a nudge from hospital administrators (the people paying the consultant's bills) will help your cause.

- *Patient satisfaction surveys and analysis*
  - Measuring patient satisfaction is important to the health and growth of your practice. Most hospitals and health care systems have computer-based systems to capture and analyze patient satisfaction information. The larger the hospital, the more complex the system. Some large systems have even purchased the expensive equipment necessary to do their own optical scanning.
  - Some of the hospital professionals who operate these huge systems are brilliant marketing researchers; professionals who can design a non-biased, well-structured statistically valid patient survey for your practice, in about an hour. They can provide technical support and even data analysis and optical scanning services during their slow periods.
  - Where can I find help with patient satisfaction surveys and other primary research? Most hospitals and health care systems have one or more professionals responsible for distributing, gathering and analyzing patient surveys. Most often these researchers work in the marketing or marketing research department. Because of the strong data analysis component of their job, you will occasionally find them in the Information Services Department.

- *Marketing advice*
  - Some hospitals and health care systems employ very talented marketing professionals who are very generous in sharing their knowledge and skill with associated medical practices. These professionals can be excellent sounding boards as your practice begins and continues to market.
  - They can give you guidance as you write your first marketing plan and offer a skilled critique of proposed promotions, ads, logos and events. Most are actively working to improve relationships with good medical practices.

Access to key individuals and populations

- *Gaining access to community leadership*
  - How many times have you heard the phrase "It's not what you know, but whom you know that counts"? There are few things as important to the growth and success of your practice as good strong relationships with the right people. Often hospitals and health care systems can provide you with an opportunity to meet, mingle and develop relationships with key community leaders, referring physicians and other individuals who can help your practice.
  - Hospitals and health care systems tend to be very well connected with the leaders within the communities they serve.   Through orchestrated events, direct community involvement and large sponsorship opportunities, hospitals find ways to gain access to key decision leaders and opinion leaders. That access can easily be shared with the right physicians and practices.
  - It's important to note that hospitals and health care systems are not likely to open this door of access to practices that are not supportive to their cause. It could be rather self-defeating to do so. Access is one of the privileges restricted for those physicians who are deemed loyal.
  - Where can you go to get access to community leadership? The answer to this question varies depending on the kinds of relationships you are seeking to establish:
    - If you want to build relationships with business leaders, speak first with members of the executive, marketing or administrative teams. They are out there interacting with local business leaders on a regular basis. They can provide the easiest access to this population.
    - If you are looking to gain access to a population of potential referring physicians, work with medical staff leadership, continuing medical education, physician marketing or marketing departments.

- If you want to work more closely with government leaders, speak with the hospital's government relations department or its lobbying consultants. For smaller hospitals, you may find access to government leaders through associations like the American Hospital Association and its many statewide branches.
- If you desire more relationships with members of the wealthy, influential and philanthropic crowd, the hospital foundation may be the key to unlock that opportunity. Keep in mind that Foundation professionals tend to be among the most protective of their relationships. It is very likely that you will only gain access to their contacts if you clearly and vocally support their cause.
- It's important that you use whatever access is granted graciously and respectfully. Professional people are often more protective of important relationships than they are of their possessions.

- *High-profile medical media opportunities*
  - It takes a very special person to be a physician and a media personality. If a physician in your practice has what it takes to be a medical reporter for local or national news program, a large hospital or health care system can help them to make the right contacts with local media leadership.
  - Large hospitals spend a huge amount in the media each year and have a number of creative arrangements with local news stations. In many instances, news stations will approach hospitals and ask for recommendations of local medical experts who can perform in front of the camera.
  - Hospitals are also the first place that news stations turn when seeking an on-the-spot medical expert for the consumer health issue of the day. If the physicians in your practice are interested in these kinds of opportunities, they would do well to make it known to the public relations, media relations and marketing managers at your local hospital.

- *Internal publications*
  - Internal hospital publications offer your physicians and your practice exposure in front of hundreds, sometimes thousands, of health care professionals. Since these publications often include valuable information for hospital and health care employees, they are well read.
  - Some of these publications offer physicians the opportunity for exposure by doing practice profiles and human-interest stories. Health care professionals represent an attractive market for a medical practice. They are among the more vocal proponents of good medical practices. If they

see or experience something they like, they will tell others. By serving this audience well, you can develop a built-in pipeline of referrals, including more health care professionals.

- Many hospitals and health care systems also have publications aimed directly at members of the medical staff. These publications can prove to be of value as a start to your physician-to-physician marketing and communications efforts.

Shared economies of scale

- *Cooperative advertising*
  - Some hospitals and health care systems offer physicians an opportunity to advertise cooperatively. In other words, the hospital and the practice share costs and share an advertising message that demonstrates unity and mutual support between the hospital and physicians.
  - Practices can benefit from the huge volume discounts that the hospital gets on advertising production and media buys. However, the hospital partner in the ads often overshadows participating physicians. Cooperative advertising can be of great value when your hospital partner is well known and respected. On the other hand, you should remember that some practices have tied themselves inextricably to a hospital partner that ended up playing the part of the villain on "60 Minutes."
  - If you choose to explore cooperative advertising, use the following guidelines:
    - Know the your hospital partner well.
    - Put the entire arrangement in writing
    - List clearly what each party contributes and how each party benefits.
    - Ensure that your physicians have a say in the final product. Whenever possible, take active control of your practice's image and exposure.
    - Make sure you have an out-clause in your contract. Protect the interests of your practice.
    - Always keep your reputation detachable from that of the hospital—just in case.

- *Physician referral services*
  - Unless you operate the only practice within a specific geographic region or your physicians have certain skills that are extremely rare in your community, you will not get a significant volume of patients from hospital-run physician referral services. Most practices are lucky to get

five patient referrals a month from even the best-promoted physician referral lines. However, by developing a good rapport with managers of these computer-based telemarketing functions, you can increase your practice's exposure and volume of patients.

- I've seen this done extremely well by a large multispecialty cancer practice that armed the physician referral team with informational pamphlets (the topics included "The seven warning signs of cancer," "Ten ways to avoid skin cancer," "Eating healthy," "Fighting cancer," among others.) They were full of information and each was emblazoned with the practice's logo. Physician referral staff used these tools so frequently that they had to call the practice to restock their supply after only a month. Yet another example of a win-win situation initiated by a medical practice.

- ### *Exposure through hospital-promoted events*
    - Health care organizations love community events. Most hold several every year. Try to select the events that will put your physicians and your practice in front of the right audience. Find out the kind of services, promotion and staffing to be provided for the event.
    - The best-attended events are the product of good content, great location, good communication and aggressive, targeted promotion. Done well, these events can be excellent exposure vehicles for your practice. On the other hand, events that are poorly organized, ill targeted and poorly attended can be very frustrating and a waste of time.
    - Before your physicians agree to participate in a hospital event, ask the following questions:
        - How does the hospital intend to attract attendees? (media, PR, advertising)
        - How many attendees are expected? How many are relevant to our specialty?
        - What other exhibitors and professionals will be working the event?
        - What is the specific role that our physicians will be playing at this event?
        - Will the physicians or practice be mentioned by name in the promotion of this event?
        - Will signage at the event include the name of the physicians or the practice?
        - Can we make our practice and personal brochures available to the event attendees?

- Will the hospital provide a supply of relevant and useful promotional premiums/give-away items?
- Have you held this event in previous years? How did it go? How was attendance?
- Select your events carefully and don't hesitate to ask for opportunities to promote the practice and physicians. It must be a mutually beneficial arrangement.

- *Making a speaker's bureau work for your practice*
  - Many hospitals and health care systems operate physician speaker's bureaus in an effort to build exposure and goodwill toward their organizations and their physicians. If your physicians have charisma and are good public speakers, your practice can find huge benefits from participating in the well-organized, hospital-based speaker's bureau.
  - Keep the following advice in mind when you consider a speaker's bureau opportunity:
    - Make sure that you are being exposed to decent size audiences (30+) that are relevant to your practice.
    - Ask how the speaker's bureau is promoted.
    - Ask if the hospital will send an invitation to a list of people supplied by your practice. These could be potential referring physicians, community leaders, media or simply personal guests. It's always good to request the opportunity to invite your own guests.
    - Ask if your practice can have a copy of the mailing list of the audience. You may find great benefit from sending follow-up information to people who were interested enough to attend. It's a good second step toward a long-term relationship.
    - Since it is a hospital-sponsored event, let them help by supplying slides, presentation support, audiovisual support, and top quality audiovisual equipment. Good resources can make the difference between a good presentation and a great presentation.
    - Make sure that your physicians are well prepared. Practice, practice, practice.

Figure 8-a

Making focus groups work for you

I worked with one OB/GYN group whose timing was extraordinary. It seemed as though they were psychic. Every time we scheduled a focus group composed of pregnant women, their office manager approached a member of the hospital marketing research team within days of the session (sometimes within hours of the session). She asked if we would mind tagging on a couple of questions to our next focus group session or test a new service concept or a logo. They tapped into our capabilities extremely well, without wearing out their welcome. Their approach was simple: "You are gathering this very targeted audience anyway. We are friends of the organization who would benefit from your help in this area." They understood that it was simple for an experienced focus group facilitator to shift gears during a session or to add a few short- answer questions to the agenda. The difficulty for the hospital or facilitator is very low—yet the benefit to the practice was quite high.

Figure 8-b

Sample Corporate Presentation Kit

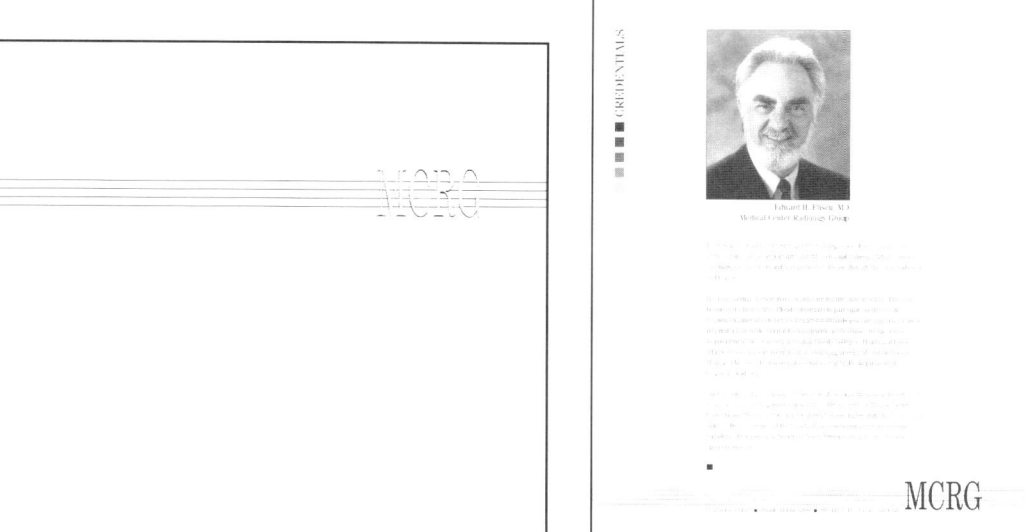

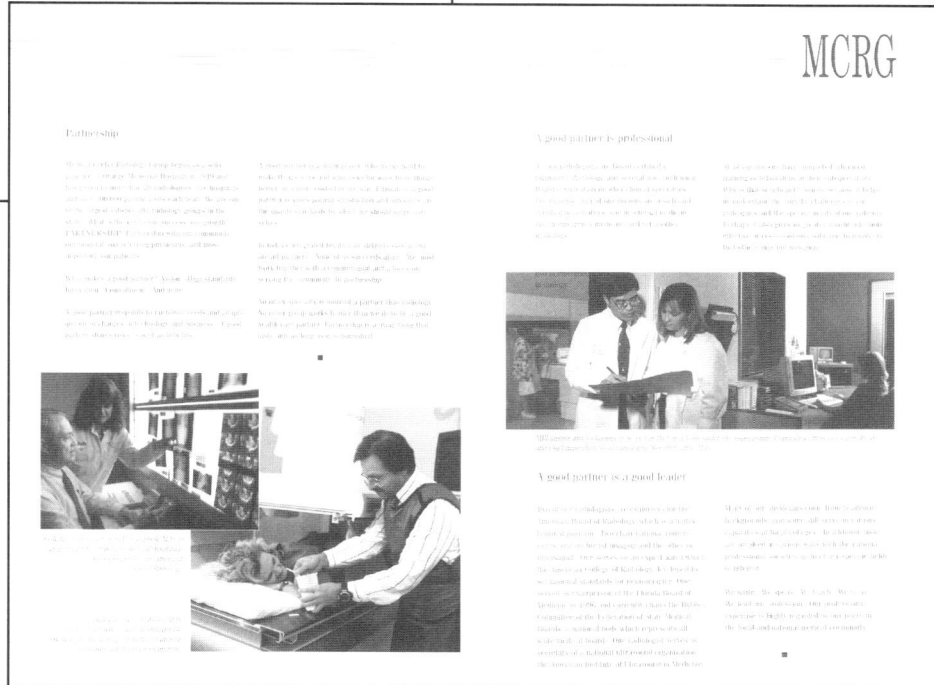

Case Study: Radiology Group

Medical Center Radiology Group is a 27-physician group practice, which is hospital based in Orlando Florida and celebrating the 50 years of imaging care. This leadership group of radiologists work exclusively at the Orlando Regional Healthcare System.

In 1984, Orlando Regional Healthcare System made the decision to build a Children's Hospital. They were looking for physicians to partner with them and to support the need for such a hospital. The support was not only that of partnering with the medical staff but also a philanthropic partnership. Medical Center Radiology Group was one of the first physician practices to make a very large contribution toward the Children's Hospital. They have continued this behavior because MCRG believes they should lead by example. They believe they should support Healthcare innovations that benefit the community.

While they have been contributing financially to the Medical Center Foundation for 15 years, the radiology group felt that they had not received appropriate recognition for their donations. This then became a marketing and branding opportunity for Medical Center Radiology Group.

In 1998, the Orlando Regional Health System made the decision to build a debt-free cancer hospital on the campus. They'd been providing cancer care for many years and now it was time to consolidate cancer efforts on one site for the enhancement of patient care.

The radiology group made a corporate decision to contribute $500,000 over five years to the new cancer center. Although the gift would be made in the group's name, each radiologist writes a personal check. However this time Medical Center Radiology Group wanted to be involved in the design of the donor recognition plan.

Goal

The goal was to position Medical Center Radiology Group positively as strong, innovative and committed physician leaders within the central Florida community and within Orlando Regional Healthcare System.

Challenge

The challenge was to create top-of-mind awareness in appropriate recognition of Medical Center Radiology Group's philanthropic endeavors, specifically as they related to Orlando Regional Healthcare System and the cancer center.

Medical Center Radiology Group, which began as a solo practice at the hospital in 1949, now has 27 physicians and covers six hospitals in four counties and cares for almost half a million patients a year.

The group has a philosophy for success: Partnership. The group is committed to education and supports patients, community-based outreach organizations and charitable foundations. The group believes that the future of Healthcare is dependent upon a strong environment, not just technology. To provide excellent patient care, they will support the family, community and Healthcare system, not just today but for the future.

All radiologists within their group are board certified and several have certification in other clinical specialties:
- Four are board certified in pediatrics;
- One is board certified in internal medicine;
- Two are board certified in emergency medicine;
- One is board certified in urology;
- Three are board certified in nuclear medicine;
- Two are radiologist examiners for the American College of Radiology;
- Two chair national meetings;
- Two chair national conferences;
- One serves on an expert panel of the American College of Radiology to set national standards for neuro imaging;
- One is treasurer of the American Institute of Ultrasound Medicine;
- One has served as chairperson of the Florida Board of Medicine;
- One serves on the Health System Board of Directors;
- One is past president of the hospital Foundation Board;
- One chairs physician fund-raising for the Cancer Center; and
- One chairs the bylaws committee of the Federation of state medical boards.

Medical Center Radiology Group has a philanthropic history:
- The radiology department of the Children's Hospital is dedicated to the group because of its financial gift;

- The third-floor of the Hubbard House, a residence for out-of-town patients' families, is dedicated to the group as a result of their gift;
- The group provides volunteers and financial support for the Special Olympics;
- The group volunteer services and has donated an x-ray machine to the local Coalition for the Homeless;
- The group has spent almost $100,000 in technologist training and education via the Medical Center Radiology Group Education Foundation;
- The group has donated in excess of $655,000 to the Orlando Regional Healthcare System Foundation; and
- Medical Center Radiology Group physicians serve on the boards of the local chapters of the United Cerebral Palsy of Central Florida, Women Playing for T.I.M.E. and Champions for Children.

Positioning benefits as a result of the large gift:
- The gift will assist in the financial development of the specialized medical institution, the Cancer Center;
- The contribution provides an opportunity for Medical Center Radiology Group to be recognized for its service to the community; and
- The gift will create an opportunity for the medical staff and administrators of Orlando Regional Healthcare System to recognize the efforts and contributions of Medical Center Radiology Group.

Targets to educate about MCRG's role in the cancer center:
- Orlando Regional Healthcare System Foundation officials and administrators;
- Cancer center officials and administrators;
- Cancer center medical staff;
- Referring physicians;
- Current and potential patients;
- Community influencers; and
- Media.

Objectives
- To generate appropriate newsworthy recognition for Medical Center Radiology Group's sizable gift to the Cancer Center;
- To demonstrate Medical Center Radiology Group's commitment to Orlando Regional Healthcare System and its philanthropic efforts;

- To recognize the involvement of Medical Center Radiology Group staff (clinical and non-clinical) in helping make this contribution possible; and
- To challenge other physician groups to get involved in the community's philanthropic endeavors.

Research and planning
- Identify an appropriate location for the announcement event;
- Identify list of all target audiences to be invited to the anncuncement event; and
- Identify an appropriate date for Medical Center Radiology Group staff ceremony.

Positioning
- Capitalize on Medical Center Radiology Group's long-term philanthropic history and involvement in the community;
- Capitalize on Medical Center Radiology Group's long-term relationship with Orlando Regional Healthcare System Foundation; and
- Capitalize on the professional expertise and experience of Medical Center Radiology Group's clinical staff.

Marketing strategies
- Host a celebratory announcement event, like an after-work cocktail party in an appropriate location off the hospital campus;
- Publicly announce that Medical Center Radiology Group is dedicating the gift in honor of its staff, both clinical and non-clinical;
- Publicly announce that the "learning center" within the Cancer Center will be named for the Medical Center Radiology Group;
- Present a larger-than-life check during this event to Foundation officials;
- Enlarge photos from the MCRG brochure and place on easels around the room;
- Play a six-minute video about Medical Center Radiology Group's role in cancer care and in its philanthropic endeavors;
- Write and distribute an appropriate news release to the media;
- Query the media about covering the contribution with the following story ideas:
  - "Docs who are different," highlighting a group of successful radiologists who have chosen to commit to the Foundation rather than increase their salaries;
  - A group practice that has quietly donated more than $1 million to the hospital;

- The group which is on the cutting edge of medical technology, that is also giving back to its community;
- A physician group who has the vision to dedicate the first year's gift to its staff who helped them become successful; and
- Profiles on the group's partners who have become leaders in the medical community.

Other strategies to consider:
- Honor Medical Center Radiology Group staff and boost morale while limiting distractions in the work environment;
- Send a personal letter to every clinical and non-clinical employee, informing them that the $500,000 gift donated by the Medical Center Radiology Group to the Cancer Center has been done so in their honor;
- This letter should be written and signed by the managing partner of the Medical Center Radiology Group; and
- It should be delivered on the same day to all employees in all six practice sites.

Outcomes:
The media department of the hospital agreed to underwrite the cost of producing and editing the six-minute videotape focusing on MCRG and its role in philanthropy and its role in cancer care. This video was presented for the first time at the cocktail party when the donation was announced.

This video has been used for fund-raising with other physician groups. The teaming of the Foundation and the medical center in using this video highlighting MCRG has positioned the group with multiple new audiences. The Medical Center Radiology Group used this video to highlight angio/interventional radiology, pediatric radiology, nuclear medicine and MRI. It allowed viewers to realize all of the roles in which radiologists play a part with referring physicians and patients.

A cocktail party was held in a private club located close to the hospital campus. Leaders in the business community, referring physicians, professional leaders in the community, bankers, accountants, hospital administrators, chamber representatives and local legislators were invited to the event. The Foundation staff created and mailed the invitations and took RSVPs for the event.

During the event, brief speeches were given by the health system CEO, president of the Cancer Center and the managing partner of the radiology group.

The *Orlando Business Journal* wrote a feature article about the gift in its health care section. In addition, the Foundation wrote a full-page article about the gift in its newsletter.

The Medical Center Radiology Group has raised its branding in the marketplace both for clinical awareness and the contribution. Although the strategies were considered, MCRG decided not to select mementos, or hold a staff luncheon. It continues to be held up as a positive example of a hospital and physician group who teamed up to enhance what they provided for their community.

LETTER

August 28, 1998

To Our Valued Clinical and Non-Clinical Imaging Team:

Medical Center Radiology Group is getting ready to celebrate 50 years of radiology care in our community. We are very proud of the quality of care we provide patients, the support we offer families, our partnerships with referring physicians and the collaborative approach we have with employers and managed care. We expect these relationships to be at the highest level.

As radiologists we realize and value that we also team with you. It is the responsibility of each and every one of you to provide your best in every patient/family interaction. It is for that reason we have decided to dedicate our gift to the Joe Lewis Institute, MD Anderson Cancer Center Orlando in your honor.

Medical Center Radiology Group has dedicated our donation of $500,000 as a tribute to our clinical and non-clinical imaging staff. You will see this reflected at the naming of the Patient Resource Center within the Joe Lewis Institute. All patients, family and staff who use this area will see a plaque that dedicates this area to you, our staff.

We are proud of each and every one of you at all of the locations where we practice.

Thank you for your dedication.

Sincerely,

(signature)
Hedrick Rivero, MD
CEO

Chapter 9

Marketing Guidelines

"The secret of success is constancy to purpose."
— Benjamin Disraeli, Earl of Beaconsfield (1870)

Now that you've identified your customers, assessed your practice, empowered your staff and held your planning retreat—what's next? It's time to position yourself for success in the marketplace. Time to develop the strategic plan that will impact how and if you will survive—your marketing plan.

Essentially, a well-written, well-implemented marketing plan is a clearly-defined blueprint that will help you fulfill your goal. It will define such elements as:

- Your market position;
- Analysis of local demographic statistics and trends;
- Analysis of your competitors;
- Strengths of your practice;
- Weaknesses of the practice;
- Opportunities available to the practice;
- Threats to the practice;
- Specific objectives of the practice;
- Evaluation of the appropriateness of the mission of the practice;
- Goals of the group;
- Strategies to achieve the goals;
- Tactics to achieve the strategies;
- Implementation responsibilities;
- Timeline for action steps; and
- Budget.

As your marketing plan evolves, you'll realize that marketing encompasses a variety of functions. For example, it should include market research, a collection of information about your group's internal and external environment. It also should include market planning, which is the framework for identifying, collecting and capturing select segments in your marketplace.

Finally, your marketing plan must include market strategy development, which will enable you to focus on new service development as well as the necessary actions that will allow you to take advantage of the opportunities and gaps in the marketplace.

Your marketing plan also may include public relations, community relations, recruitment, internal marketing, patient liaison and contracting. In addition, marketing should be integrated with other management systems, such as operations, finance and clinical quality issues.

A very simple marketing plan will have the following components:
- Description of the target market:
  - Age;
  - Sex;
  - Profession;
  - Income level;
  - Education level;
  - Zip code;
- Market research data;
- Direct and indirect competitors;
- Description of competitors;
- Strengths and weaknesses of competitors;
- Description of products and services;
- Demand for product or service;
- Description of what differentiates your products and services;
- Similarities and dissimilarities between your products and services and those of your competitors;
- Special features and selling points of your products and services;
- Goals;
- Objectives:
  - Percentages to be achieved;
  - Measurement guide;
- Strategies:
  - Description of what group must do to achieve goals;

- Tactics:
  - Steps to implement strategies;
- Marketing budget:
  - Costs allocated for public relations, marketing, advertising and promotions; and
  - Advertising media and estimated cost of placement.

Marketing through branding

As noted before, your brand is your personality. Thus, it deserves serious consideration. It can be a name, design, symbol or mark which enhances the value of your practice beyond its functional purpose—something that distinguishes you from others. Your brand makes a promise. A strong brand is trustworthy and possesses great value. It has meaning, prestige and presence, and it helps confirm what is expected.

Quite simply, branding means developing brand name identity or image positioning. It's the process by which you establish and maintain the unique identity that triggers immediate recognition and (you hope) a positive image whenever your name is seen or heard. It's also the type of awareness which predisposes patients and others to choose your practice over another.

Over time, the added value that accrues from branding is referred to as brand equity. This includes such assets as consumer awareness, perceived quality and willingness to purchase your product or use your service. In health care, this translates into a willingness to choose to be a loyal patient, to speak highly of the practice and refer others for reasons of patient advocacy, concern and clinical expertise.

Branding allows you to build awareness by creating a clear image and recognition for your group. It helps make your patients feel secure and confident that they have selected the right practice for their health care.

However, for a brand to be effective, users must be aware of it. They also must believe it provides a benefit that they want or need, and they must find its performance to be superior to other similar products or services. In short, users must develop a relationship with the brand which makes them feel good about selecting it and continuing to use it. The key to this is consistent, effective marketing.

If you position your practice as unique and as the answer to your patients' needs, you must market your group's image (brand) so patients, referring physicians, and managed care payers will do business with you.

Is branding necessary in today's managed care marketplace? Definitely. Although it's true that provider choices are often limited, that doesn't mean that branding can be ignored. In heavily competitive markets, it's more important than ever for leaders to develop and sustain their unique image and identity—their brand. This makes it more difficult for competitors to attract new market share by offering new products or services or perceived product or service improvements.

By raising your level of awareness with specific target audiences, you communicate who you are, what you stand for, and your commitment to serve your community. In addition, it is your responsibility to make sure that your customers recognize and can find you. The tools used to accomplish these goals include:

Development and use of a distinctive logo/graphic identity;
- Development of community partnerships;
- Alignment with power centers;
- Patient education;
- Development of one-on-one relationships with major employers;
- Active involvement with business coalitions; and
- Development of positive relations with print, electronic and radio media.

Long-term, consistent use of these vital tools will help position your practice for long-term success through branding.

Research shows, for example, that the desire to select the best brand increases when a family experiences health care urgency. The brand of a community cancer center is not particularly relevant to a family under usual circumstances. But if a family member is diagnosed with cancer, that same family becomes much more sensitive as it goes "shopping" for the best brand available to them.

Branding for medical practices is mostly about building trust between patients, physicians and other community leaders. Obviously, it's important to maintain quality, service and access, but in addition, you must maximize existing relationships and move beyond that to those things that matter most to your target audiences.

In today's health care environment, building your brand through marketing helps you control your own destiny. However, it means you no longer can avoid change or even maintain the status quo. You must develop and implement strategies that meet—or exceed—the needs and expectations of your customers.

How do you accomplish this goal? Look around your community and ask yourself how you can offer "added value" to your customers. Look for ways to set your own strategic focus, to lead the market rather than follow your competitors. Offer products and services that provide a quantum leap in value for your customers and your community. Although this may require additional resources—both human and monetary—it is a valuable investment that will pay off handsomely as it positions your practice positively in the marketplace.

To review what has already been emphasized earlier in this book, the most important element of this goal is to identify and understand your customers, along with their stated, as well as unstated and unmet, needs. Then, meet those needs in ways that extend beyond your ordinary offering of products and services.

In addition to knowing your customers, you also must know your competitors. It is not sufficient to know what old or new competitors are doing now. Figure out what they intend to do tomorrow so strategies can be developed to combat them. This can be accomplished effectively by conducting an intensive competitive review and sharing that information during quarterly Board management meetings.

It's also important to know yourself, as discussed in Chapter 4. Ask questions— and listen to what you hear. Have the cultural values that draw employees and inspire extraordinary performance been compromised? Is there divisiveness within the operating team? Cynicism, indifference, negativity and defensiveness can destroy even the strongest organization. What does close observation of actual behavior, confidential interviews and cultural audits illustrate about the spirit of the organization? Remember, if those in leadership positions are not vested in the vision of the practice, potentially significant information may be missed because those looking at it will do so through traditional, selfish, greedy or non-motivated lenses.

Also, you should promote brainstorming by your entire group. Approach all ideas with a conceptual vision—and then figure out how to make them work. Think of products and services as a connection to multiple customers, not simply as a means to reimbursement.

During a strategic retreat, for example, the ideas offered may be so powerful and radical that they redefine the focus for the future. Ideas should be offered, not because they will be financially successful, but because they will make a difference to customers. If you can achieve that, financial success is sure to follow.

Finally, question the norm. Look for ways to turn information into ideas for action. Identify real insights which work toward preventing future disasters, creating new contracts, investing in new technologies, shifting the group's direction, addressing new markets, redesigning modes of operations and delegating responsibility.

Of course, asking unsettling questions can cause anxiety. However, it is through non-traditional thinking and dynamic tension that innovative value is discovered. Out of this can come creative and innovative marketing and communication strategies.

Even with the best of intentions, however, you may find yourself in a marketplace that is not durable. Remember, marketing created to build brand awareness is still effective and lasting for the group as health care goes through its next phase of development. In that case, this valuable positioning is already in place for use in multiple ways, depending on the next evolution of customer or partner.

Understanding media relations and using the media as a resource

Let's look closer at how positive relationships with your local media can serve as a stepping stone for achieving your goals.

Say, for example, you plan to introduce a new product or service in your marketplace. One of the most effective vehicles you can use to deliver your message is the media—electronic (television), radio and print. Although you'll also use other methods of reaching your audience—direct mail, sponsorships, partnering, open houses, health fairs, etc.—there is tremendous power in using today's ubiquitous media.

First, it's important to communicate with your local medical reporters and make them aware of the special services or procedures your group brings to the community. It's important to think about what their needs are and prepare your approach to assist them in doing their jobs.

Here are several important steps you can take to position your practice effectively:
- Define what your group or a specific physician has to offer that is of special interest to your community.
- Is this a new service in your area?
- Are there limited physicians who are credentialed to perform this procedure?
- Is there a special interest story that has broad appeal?
- Is there a demographic group that will be especially interested in this health care procedure—such as—teenagers, mothers of toddlers, menopausal

women, seniors, golfers, ballroom dancers, women of child-bearing age or
weekend warrior athletes?

- Do you have a physician who is willing to cooperate with the medical
reporter?
- Is your physician flexible to meet the time frame of the reporter or the
medical producer?
- Do you have a relationship with your patient base that will provide a patient
willing to go on camera about his or her health care issue?

Using radio to tell your story

As you're developing marketing strategies, there also are times when purchasing
media will be the most appropriate and effective way to get your message to the
market. Because radio broadcasts reach almost anyone—in homes, cars, offices and
retail businesses—radio can be a powerful, yet financially efficient marketing tool for
group practices. Radio can be used effectively to tell a story, call to action and
control a message—all in good taste. In fact, during radio's highest-rated hours
(morning and afternoon drive times), it draws a larger audience than television in
many cities.

When researching the best methods for reaching target markets, it is important to set
up appointments with the sales representatives from several radio stations in your
community. As part of their jobs, these reps collect excellent demographic
information and frequently, can be very creative in preparing a proposal to show
how radio can help you work toward reaching your goals.

Usually, each station attracts a very tightly defined audience. Since the stations tend
to do aggressive marketing research, they are very aware of the demographic,
geographic, psychographic and cultural characteristics of their listening audiences.
Thus, by meeting with various station reps, your group can match its patient and
community target audiences—assuring that advertising dollars are spent effectively.

Here's an example that illustrates this process. During a strategic retreat, a large
orthopaedic group had established goals that would allow them to achieve their
vision. One of those goals was to remain positioned as leaders in total joint
replacement and be considered the practice of choice when a patient decided to
have surgery. One of their strategies was to reach the young senior market, those 55
years of age and older.

Many tactics were developed to achieve their year-long campaign of positioning as
total joint leaders in their market. One of these tactics involved purchasing time for

a radio campaign. As the budget was limited, the group decided to stay with one station and go for frequency and reach with that station. It was felt that they would have better penetration to the radio market with that approach. The station they selected helped them match their target audience to particular programming. The station also volunteered to produce their ad spot at no cost.

A copywriter was retained to write three 60-second health informational commercials. These spots focused on an awareness of pain and discomfort from arthritic joints. They encouraged listeners to discuss options with their personal family physician. However, if the option indicated the need for a total joint replacement, the listener was encouraged to call this orthopaedic group for printed health care information. Because of the demographics of the marketplace, the phone number was offered in Spanish as well as in English.

The group was very lucky as it planned this campaign. One patient had been a television talent in the community for many years. Although now retired, he was still an icon among seniors. The administrator called the patient and asked if he would be interested in being the voice of the radio spots. He was delighted to participate in a professional role and agreed to go to the radio station and work with the station team to produce the spots.

The bonus for the group was to have the former television star's trusted soothing voice tell the message. The group provided him with a one-time honorarium for his work that was appropriate for radio talent. This was greatly appreciated by the patient and showed respect for his talent. Many patients commented to the orthopaedic surgeons that they had heard the ad and remembered it, not only for the message, but also because of the delivery by the retired television anchor who was perceived as a friend by the community.

To track responses, the group used a selected telephone extension that was noted in the commercial. Each day, the message center was checked and callers were mailed informational fact sheets on total joint replacement. In addition, as a promotional item, the fact sheets were packaged in a health record file folder which was given to patients to hold their medical records. The feedback was that this was appreciated and considered very useful by older patients who see several physicians in a year. The medical record file was branded with the group's logo, phone number and 800 number.

By the way, this radio campaign was so successful that the same story line was used to create a similar one for television. A 30-second commercial, narrated by the same retired television anchor, was produced and subsequently scheduled on the top-rated local television station. It also received positive feedback and increased business for the group.

One of the advantages of using radio as a vehicle to share your message is the low cost, both to create commercials and to purchase airtime. While prices differ in every market, you can expect a 60-second spot to range between $40 and $250 during peak times. Depending on the frequency and reach you need, you should negotiate the best rate with your ad rep and build this expense into your total marketing budget.

Your group can write a spot or have one written exclusively for you. The radio announcer can read it, or voice talent can be used. The station will usually help you produce a commercial, including sound effects, often at no additional charge. That is another reason to develop a relationship with your sales rep, who can be instrumental in assisting you with this element of your plan.

Public radio also accepts some sponsorships, usually at a lower cost than commercial radio. Although public radio and television do not boast the same audience size as commercial stations, sometimes their audience is exactly the target group you want to influence. Public radio often reaches more community-minded and involved people. These may be local civic leaders, board members, club presidents and people who find time to volunteer and do things in your community.

Here are a few tips that show how to get the most bang for your radio buck:
1. Define the target audience you want to reach.
2. What are you selling them?
3. What do you want them to know?
4. What is your call to action?
5. Set ad goals and a budget.
6. Keep in mind that effective radio advertising builds name, product or service recognition by repetition, so budget enough dollars for airplay.

Keep in mind that health care information and experiences can be very confusing to your patients and the public at large. You have an excellent opportunity to share information about what's happening locally, to regionalize national stories, to position yourself as a local authority and to raise the brand of your group by consistently working on the marriage between medicine and the media.

Television as an educational forum

Traditionally, televisions stations have used a journalist as the health care reporter. These on-air talents usually presented health segments at least three times a week, typically in the 5 p.m. or 5:30 p.m. slot. However, things began to change at the local level once the big three networks—NBC, ABC and CBS—hired and promoted their national talent, who just happened to be physicians.

Surveys and station feedback indicated that viewers preferred getting health care information from physicians, rather than reporters. This opened the door for local physicians to become the "talent" for health care reporting, either replacing or working with a full-time station reporter.

In the late '90s, many local television stations began to search for an on-air physician talent. In three instances, I have been retained to help local affiliate stations find a physician who could become the station's television doctor. Although there have been different parameters at each station, they basically want:

1. A well-credentialed MD or DO;

2. A physician who can enter all hospital facility boundaries for the purpose of covering a health care story;

3. A physician who is available one day a week to shoot two or three stories for airing later in the week;

4. A physician who also has time on a second day a week to work with the medical producer discussing story ideas, articles from the *Journal of the American Medical Association,* the *New England Journal of Medicine* or other publications and on-line wire services;

5. A physician who is well-connected in the health care community and who can become educated quickly in areas that may not be his/her personal area of expertise;

6. A physician who can be called upon night or day—hospital or office, home or station—if there is a national crisis or emergency that the station wants to cover for its local audience;

7. A physician who can create story ideas that are beneficial to the community;

8. A physician who will agree not to travel during ratings or sweeps periods (November, February, May and July);

9. A physician who is available for station promotions; and

10. A physician who finds the salary acceptable.

The challenge for the television stations is to find a physician who meets all of these criteria and still can stay in the good graces of his/her group. Although the television physician talent is paid a generous salary, in my experience, it is well below what the physician will earn if he/she is working as a full-time employee in the group model. At times, this has led to group concerns that the television physician was being positioned with an opportunity to become a celebrity at the expense of the group.

As a consultant to television stations and physicians, I view it somewhat differently. The television doctor will be perceived as a leader and a member of a strong group or strong practice. The television doctor has the opportunity, simply by becoming a television personality, to raise the brand of the group and the perceived quality of its physicians as a whole.

The group may argue that the television doctor isn't identified as Dr. Sherman of the Trans Medical Group, for example, but rather as Dr. Sherman, WXYZ-television. That is true. However, when viewers call in, they are referred to the physician both at the station and at the physician's practice. Naturally, this provides increased visibility for the group as a whole.

When the television physician is called upon to respond to a story or national issue in a remote setting, the doctor is encouraged to be in "medical work" attire. This often means in a lab coat with the monogram of the group on the upper left hand or pocket side. This again raises visibility and brand awareness for the group.

I once received a call from a client wanting to know if he should make himself available to the media. There was a concern that the media was out to create a controversial story and that the reporter would embarrass him.

As we discussed the opportunity, I learned that a reporter had called the practice looking for a medical authority to comment on a news item that had been on the health care wire service. Although the reporter did not know anyone specifically in the practice, she wanted to do the interview on Sentinel Node Mapping by the end of the week.

I counseled the administrator to take the call or return the call promptly. When reporters are on deadline, your goal should be to nurture positive, long-term, media relations. Make sure you understand the topic and assure the reporter you'll locate one of your surgeons who will be comfortable talking about Sentinel Node Mapping as a diagnostic tool for breast cancer evaluation.

During the initial call to the reporter or medical producer, the surgeon can lay out more than one scenario as to how he can help the reporter, and thus the station, with a medical story which is exclusive to them. The surgeon should agree to go on camera to respond to the immediate story. However, he/she can propose a follow-up segment involving a patient who is undergoing Sentinel Node Mapping. The surgeon should offer the patient's permission and support to take the story to the community via television news.

The surgeon also can suggest developing the story to be of more interest to the women of the community. He/she might suggest interviewing the nuclear medicine radiologist or pathologist who performs the procedure, the radiologist who reads mammography and even the oncologist who will take over care when the surgeon completes his job.

At a minimum, the television station can video the patient in the Nuclear Medicine Department as she is having her scan read by the radiologist/pathologist and the surgeon. Based on what's learned in the scan, the reporter will be able to interview the surgeon explaining to the patient what Sentinel Node Mapping has told him and how he is going to approach her surgery for breast cancer.

This is win/win situation for several health care leaders. The surgeon is positioned as leader of the team and surgeon of choice for the breast biopsy. The nuclear medicine department gains visibility as having state-of-the-art technology and equipment. The hospital is positioned as a leader that is invested in women's health, as nuclear medicine is one of the hospital's services. Finally, viewers gain a sense that breast cancer diagnosis is handled by a team of physicians working together for the benefit of the patient.

The most successful interviews hinge on the physician's understanding of the basic aim of the reporter. To make their deadline, reporters usually want to get in and out of your office or surgical suite as quickly as possible. It's to your advantage to ask reporters what type of information they are looking for and work to answer it succinctly. Because of the time limitations with television, reporters are looking for sound bites with passion and clarity.

I further counseled this administrator and surgeon to work to establish a positive, ongoing relationship with the reporter and the television station. The positioning goal for the future is to develop a working relationship with the reporter so that you will be the "go to" practice whenever there is a surgical story opportunity. The reporter will hope to come back to you in the future, and she/he will want to develop a trusting, working relationship. This being the goal, don't be afraid to pitch a story to the media. Keep in mind, however, that the story must be news, must have broad appeal and must be conveniently covered.

Another advantage is financial. If the group had to pay for this television exposure from the media, it would cost a fortune.

Here are a few recommendations that will help you position for success in dealing with the media;

- Be responsive to media calls. Make every effort to return calls personally or delegate to someone who can respond to the media within the hour. You may not be able to assist with the story on a given day, but you will keep and enhance your relationship with the medical reporter.
- Ask the reporter to define the topic and inquire if she/he could give you a few planned questions so you can think about it in advance. This is a reasonable request.
- Get to the point—the interview will be edited into short statements that tell the essence of the story. Although the interview may take 10 to 15 minutes or more, the edited story will probably be no longer than 60 to 90 seconds.
- Use clear examples and speak as basically as you would if you were talking to an eighth-grade school child. It is important to create graphic images as you speak, so that the audience can absorb the story easily and memorably.
- Avoid medical jargon. Examples are: bump instead of lesion, cut versus sever, imaging versus radiology procedures, and blood vessels rather than arteries.
- Don't fudge on your answers. You are not giving an adversarial interview. You are partnering with the reporter to bring health care information to your community. If you aren't sure of the answer, say so, then offer to research the answer and get back to the reporter.

Cosmetic surgery mini-marketing campaign

GOAL: Achieve #1 brand equity in cosmetic and reconstructive surgery in Western Florida.

CHALLENGES:
1. Strengthen internal marketing.
2. Develop a strong brand name identity.
3. Investigate new technology with market appeal.
4. Increase cosmetic volume.
5. Develop a program to maintain and protect desired managed care relations.
6. Build and maintain a strong referral physician program.
7. Expand skin care services.

MARKET POSITIONING: What can make your practice unique in the eyes of your target markets?
1. Convenient and prime location.
2. A practice which cares about patient care, quality and a sensitive environment.
3. A mature place to go for cosmetic and reconstructive care.
4. A place to go where each patient is treated as a priceless commodity.
5. A practice whose doctors regularly perform a high volume of specialized procedures with good outcomes.
6. A place to go for privacy and surgical excellence.

RESEARCH AND PLANNING:
1. Learn what resources exist within the computer software.
2. Identify and respond to appropriate community sponsorships.
3. Evaluate print materials:
   - Evaluate logo;
   - Create a mission statement;
   - Develop a practice handbook;
   - Create a presentation kit;
   - Revise physician bios and photos; and
   - Review procedure handouts.
4. Identify potential networking opportunities for the physicians.
5. Develop a list of managed care administration contact people.
6. Track outcomes of appointments booked after a video imaging appointment.
7. Identify media placement opportunities.
8. Review Yellow Page ad design.
9. Identify radio talk show opportunities.

10. Identify opportunities for targeted marketing programs.
11. Develop a system for first-year anniversary post-op appointment.
12. Develop a system for direct mailing to existing patient base.
13. Semi-annually conduct a patient satisfaction survey.
14. Identify referring practices to invite to staff wine and cheese parties.
15. Identify areas in the business community in which to become involved.

TARGET MARKETS: ___Managed care ___Employers ___Referring physicians

___Potential referrers ___All physicians ___Hospitals ___Patients

___Employees ___Employees' families ___Vendors ___Local VIPs ___Media

___Trade Associations ___Selected community groups ___General community

___Key Influencers ___Others

CHALLENGE #1

Strengthen internal marketing.

Strategy:
- Enhance print materials and strengthen image;
- Redesign logo to create a sense of warmth and nurturing;
- Create a stationery package; and
- Develop a corporate image for all print material.

Strategy:
- Create a mission statement; and
- Use mission statement on practice brochure, presentation kit and in reception area and patient rooms.

Strategy:
- Develop a practice handbook;
  - Distribute to all new and returning patients; and
  - Distribute at community talks.

Strategy: ✔
- Create a presentation folder;
  - Use with new patient letter;
  - Practice brochure;
  - Physician resumes;

Improve Patient data capture

- Patient education materials; and
- Use in select community outreach opportunities.

Strategy:
- Revise physician bios to coordinate with print image. ✓

Strategy:
- Review Yellow Page ad design.

Strategy:
- Develop a system for direct mailing to existing patient base;
  - New information;
  - New facilities;
  - Open house;
  - Group consults;
  - Educational forums; and
  - New products and services.

Strategy:
- Select a promotional item for give-a-way purposes. ✓

CHALLENGE #2

Develop a strong brand name identity.

Strategy:
- Develop a program to integrate Western Florida Plastic Surgery into the community;
- Utilize Chamber of Commerce:
  - Join WFCC;
  - Have Dr. Nice apply to Leadership Western Florida;
  - Underwrite a program in the community with women as the target audience;
- Utilize appropriate communication tools; and
- Develop corporate sponsorships.

Strategy:
- Develop a multi-media ad campaign;
- Create and place print ads;
- Investigate radio campaigns, which are service specific; and
- Produce a television ad for electronic opportunities.

Strategy:
- Take advantage of speaking opportunities:
  - Hospitals;
  - Women's groups;
  - Teen programs; and
  - Men's groups.

Strategy:
- Become involved in a community project.

CHALLENGE # 3

Investigate new technology with market appeal.

Strategy:
- Engage video imaging for 90-day trial.

Strategy
- Offer free imaging to guests at staff "wine and cheese" receptions.

Strategy
- Track consult scheduling of patients who use imaging.

Strategy
- Remain open to other new technology.

Strategy:
- Develop scripts to use during phone inquiries to encourage appointment scheduling.

CHALLENGE # 4

Increase cosmetic practice.

Strategy:
- Create ad campaigns that are procedure specific.

Strategy:
- Create print materials that assist in cross-selling.

Strategy:
- Develop relations with media reporters.

Strategy:
- Create and distribute press releases on interesting cases or technology.

Strategy:
- Develop relations with vendors who can be influencers:
  - Massage therapists;
  - Personal trainers;
  - Manicurists;
  - Lingerie salespeople; and
  - Hair dressers.

Strategy:
- Review your personal networks to offer private group consultations about new procedures.

Strategy:
- Look for opportunities to provide public speaking or participate on panels.

CHALLENGE # 5

Develop a program to maintain and protect desired managed care relations.

Strategy:
- Create a database of managed care contacts.

Strategy:
- Create a program for inviting managed care contacts to the practice.

Strategy:
- Create a database or at least a list of primary care and OB/GYN physicians on plans on which you want to maintain relations:
  - Research what is important to them;
  - Provide them with news of interest; and
  - Entertain them.

Strategy:
- Develop a philosophy and game plan for contracting with managed care.

Strategy:
- Research what role reconstructive surgery plays in managed care.

CHALLENGE # 6

Build and maintain a strong referral physician program.

Strategy:
• Continue interacting with referring physicians as is traditional.

Strategy:
• Create a physician survey to find out how well you're doing.

Strategy:
• Develop a program to respond to new physicians entering the market:
    • Develop a method for collecting information;
    • Develop a database;
    • Provide personal attention when possible;
    • Send a welcome letter; and
    • After a meeting or a personal phone call, send a presentation kit and include services, products and openings for new patients.

Strategy:
• Develop and look for opportunities to interact with the physician community.

Strategy:
• When appropriate by specialty, send cosmetic or reconstructive articles that will be of interest.

Strategy:
• Develop a campaign to meet all OB/GYN physicians:
    • Have a front-office party;
    • Host a social event; and
    • Offer to do a joint seminar to their patients, which involves both specialties.

CHALLENGE #7

Expand skin care services.

Strategy:
• Create a campaign to communicate about skin care issues to existing patients.

Strategy:
- Create a fact sheet for presentation kit.

Strategy:
- Develop relations with vendors who can be influencers:
  - Massage therapists;
  - Spas;
  - Estheticians;
  - Personal trainers;
  - Manicurists;
  - Lingerie salespeople; and
  - Hair dressers.

Strategy:
- Create a media interest in your skin care approach.

Strategy:
- Author an article for small local publications.

Strategy:
- Continue to maintain interest in all patients no matter what procedure they have.

Strategy:
- Develop mail order or phone order ease of product purchases.

Case Study: Orthopaedic "Milk Mustache"

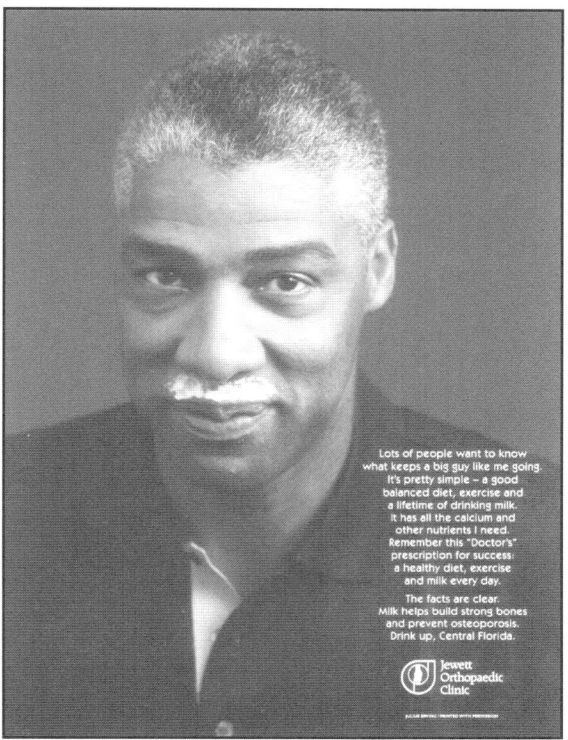

Lots of people want to know what keeps a big guy like me going. It's pretty simple – a good balanced diet, exercise and a lifetime of drinking milk. It has all the calcium and other nutrients I need. Remember this "Doctor's" prescription for success: a healthy diet, exercise and milk every day.

The facts are clear. Milk helps build strong bones and prevent osteoporosis. Drink up, Central Florida.

Jewett Orthopaedic Clinic

In 1998, the Jewett Orthopaedic Clinic in Orlando, FL, implemented an innovative advertising campaign in conjunction with the NBA Orlando Magic basketball team. A unique–and creative—extension of the practice's traditional campaign, which is placed each year to promote the team physicians, this special group of ads was tied directly to the popular national "Got Milk?" campaign.

The series of ads featured Magic team personnel wearing the now familiar "mustache" with copy appropriate to the individual's position with the team. It also featured information about how milk builds strong bones with a tie-in to orthopaedics and how Jewett helps athletes and others maintain good orthopaedic health. Although the local ads did not use the milk logo or slogan, they were used with the permission of the national campaign organizers.

Armed with the elusive "recipe" for the milk mustache shown in the popular national ads featuring celebrities, Jewett photographed Orlando Magic personnel such as "Dr. J," otherwise known as Julius Erving, sporting an identical mustache. Six ads were produced, each using a different personality.

The objective of the campaign was: To produce an eye-catching, distinctive four-color ad series which would attract the attention of sports fans throughout Central Florida, while promoting a broader message—that Jewett Orthopaedic Clinic can diagnose and treat sports-related injuries as well as other orthopaedic problems of all types.

As an extension of the ad campaign, the group partnered with the Dairy Council and the National Osteoporosis Foundation to co-sponsor the 1998 Better Bones Tour, a national program that takes the Milk Mustache Mobile on an annual tour across the country. Orlando was one of some 100 city stops on the tour.

The goal of the Better Bones Tour was to educate Americans about bone health and promote the benefits of drinking milk. In addition, this special event features a consumer milk mustache contest (with a chance to win an appearance in *People Magazine*), which features free bone-density screenings and educational materials on the importance of drinking three glasses of milk a day for calcium and better bone health.

Jewett also offered educational material from its special promotional booth at the site. In 1999-2000, the Better Bones Tour expanded to become known as the Cruise for Calcium. This was done to expand risk awareness screenings and health information to include blood pressure and colon cancer in addition to osteoporosis. Thus, it made the event more valuable to men and women.

As a result of its involvement in 1998, Jewett was invited to participate as a co-sponsor during the Orlando visit. Jewett determined that this event was big enough to bring in an additional partner. Building on its relationships, the practice partnered with the NBA Orlando Magic to bring the Cruise for Calcium Tour with the Milk Mustache Mobile to a Sunday game at the Orlando Arena.

The Milk Mobile set up three hours before the game, which gave Jewett and the Cruise for Calcium Tour exposure to 17,000 people attending a Sunday afternoon basketball game.

Jewett's marketing also included a publicity tie-in with a local television station to promote the local visit of the Cruise for Calcium Milk Mobile. With the cooperation of the Dairy Farmers, the Clinic was able to provide film footage and osteoporosis data to the station's health reporter to be used in a locally targeted news story about the tour. The reporter focused the story on osteoporosis and the need to increase calcium in our diets. She included the information about the bone-density and blood-pressure testing machines, along with the *People Magazine* milk contest.

This campaign provided extensive, positive visibility for Jewett. In fact, the Milk Mustache photos using local celebrities was so successful, Jewett was also able to get permission to use the same strategy for the University of Central Florida ad campaign. This series of ads featured the University President, the Athletic Director, the Football and Baseball Coaches and the University's most famous alumni athlete and Olympic Gold medal soccer player, Michele Akers.

As a result of this campaign, Jewett achieved the following:
- Enhanced brand name identity;
- An opportunity to do relationship marketing;
- A strong memorable campaign that has lasted 24 months; and
- An opportunity to align with other power centers.

10

How Successful Practices Market

"Competitive edge comes from a better ability to live in the fog of reality and make rapid, excellent interpretations of where the world is at this moment, and where it is headed."

—- Warren Bennis, leadership guru

Marketing plan of action example 1: Allergy practice

In the late '90s, we worked with a six-person allergy practice in Tennessee whose goal was to become the premier allergy and asthma group in its community and in surrounding areas. This practice had a managing partner who frequently attended conferences and seminars that focus on practice management. She worked closely with the practice administrator and listened to recommendations about how to position the practice for the future.

One physician within the practice understood the power of the media and enjoyed serving as spokesperson for the practice. She made herself available on a range of topics relating to allergy and asthma, and became the media expert for allergy topics within the community.

Following a strategic practice retreat, this group decided to develop a written marketing plan. The group provided all the background information, but because of perceived budgetary restraints, no formal market research was performed (not an ideal situation). Fortunately, while developing the plan, we were able to identify important market trends and provide general recommendations to respond to these trends.

Although this community had minimal managed care penetration at the time, the group wanted to be informed about the subject as it looked toward the future. The retreat and development of the marketing plan were designed to help the group establish a positioning vision for the future. As discussed in earlier chapters, it is important to conduct a situational analysis and understand the trends in your marketplace prior to developing your marketing plan.

Let's take a look at this group's plan.

Strategic Marketing Plan of Action
for the
Tennessee Allergy & Asthma Center
(Campaign to position center for the future)

Marketing overview

The key to positioning Tennessee Allergy and Asthma Center in the next 24 to 36 months is to differentiate from other allergy and asthma competitors in the marketplace. This can be accomplished by taking maximum advantage of the "value-added" and other differentiating factors that substantiate why others should do business with Tennessee Allergy and Asthma Center.

Consider adopting a theme positioning Tennessee Allergy and Asthma Center as "Your community partners for allergy and asthma care." This should be used consistently in all promotional and marketing materials.

In addition, Tennessee Allergy and Asthma Center must make a commitment to move forward on the recommended strategies and tactics in this plan and to provide the budget to accomplish these tasks. You should use this plan as an overall road map to affect change within your practice, realizing that it is a fluid document, not one cast in concrete. It is a living plan of action that merely provides the infrastructure that you need to move forward toward success. As such, it is important that you respond as necessary to changes as they occur.

Finally, you must track your efforts by following through on implementation and demanding accountability. It is recommended that you review your efforts every 90 days and proceed based on what has been accomplished at that point.

MARKETING GOAL

- To achieve number one brand equity in allergy and asthma services throughout our community
    Brand equity = awareness + usage + perceived quality

MARKETING OBJECTIVES

- Increase net revenues in 1998-99 by (TBD) percent;
- Increase number of referrals in 1998-99 by (TBD) percent;
- Increase number of referring physicians in 1998-99 by (TBD) percent;
- Increased presence on managed care panels in 1998 99 by (TBD) percent;
- Increase patient satisfaction in 1998-99 by (TBD) percent; and
- Increase branding identity in 1998-99 by (TBD) percent.

(TBD = to be determined)

TARGET MARKETS

- Referring physicians;
- Managed care plans;
- Coalitions;
- Employers;
- Internal staff;
- Patients;
- Corporate community; and
- Media.

MARKET POSITIONING

Market positioning asks the question, "What makes your practice unique in the eyes of your target markets?" The following factors were identified at the strategic retreat:

- Convenient locations;
- A practice that cares about its patients, quality and a sensitive environment;
- An innovative place to go for allergy and asthma care;
- A practice whose doctors regularly perform a high volume of specialized procedures with good outcomes; and
- A ten-year involvement in clinical trials.

Obviously, there are many other differentiating characteristics that shou d be considered when determining your unique position or the value-added factors that can be used to set the Tennessee Allergy and Asthma Center apart from its competitors. These must be identified and used as you implement this plan. Remember:

Value is:
The worth of a thing in money or goods at a certain time or market price;

The quality of something according to which it is thought of as being desirable, useful, etc. A fair or proper equivalent in money, commodities, etc.

$$\text{Value} = \frac{\text{Access x Service x Quality}}{\text{Cost}}$$

Therefore:

- If you increased access, you increase value;
- If you increase service, you increase value;
- If you increase quality, you increase value; and
- If you decrease cost, you increase value.

CHALLENGES (strategies)

There are six primary challenges that the Tennessee Allergy and Asthma Center should address to achieve success in its marketing campaign. These are:

- Strengthen internal relations;
- Develop and maintain a strong brand identity;
- Maintain and protect desired managed care relations;
- Build and maintain a strong referral physician program;
- Build brand name identity with major employers; and
- Enhance patient relations.

TACTICS (by challenges)

CHALLENGE # 1

- **Strengthen internal relations:**
  - *Strategy: Review all print materials.*

  - *Strategy: Promote your mission:*
    - Create a clear, concise mission statement and use it on all your communication materials, including your patient handbook and a presentation piece for managed care contacts and referring physicians in your community. Also, incorporate your theme ("Your community partners for allergy and asthma care") into your mission statement and post it in your reception areas, business office and clinical patient areas.

  - *Strategy: Determine all your value-added advantages:*
    - Review the value-added benefits your group brings to the community and to all the customers, patients, clients and partners with whom you do business, and which you identified during your retreat. Determine if

these are still valid and if others should be added. Those already identified include:
- Special expertise and asthma treatment;
- High-quality allergy care;
- Multiple locations with new facilities;
- Good control of asthma which lowers absences from work and school;
- Choice of male and female physicians;
- Years of clinical trials involving new pharmaceutical products which benefit national research and your patients; and
- Commitment to patient education.
- Commit this list of factors to writing and use for all appropriate opportunities, such as on your communication materials.

- *Strategy: Educate your staff about changes in the health care environment by in-service meetings held twice a year on this topic:*
  - Invite managed care director, health care coalition leader and hospital administrator to explain the health care situation from each of their viewpoints; and
  - Have a health care attorney conduct a presentation on compliance and fraud and abuse.

- *Strategy: Conduct an annual staff retreat:*
  - Staff retreats are an essential part of any smooth running office and indirectly, can contribute greatly to patient satisfaction;
  - Conducting a retreat gives employees a voice in the design of the systems that allow the office to function properly. It also gives them more "buy-in" to the future of the practice. By holding a retreat and allowing staff to have input, you let them know that they are appreciated as employees and their opinions are appreciated as well. They do their jobs every day, so they may be able to come up with efficient, more effective systems that will help the practice be more cost-effective and service-oriented in today's market;
  - This is an especially important tactic for Tennessee Allergy and Asthma Center because of the recent reorganization of your front office staff. Providing a retreat allows your staff to focus on the positive side of your practice; it will benefit all involved; and
  - For your small staff, a "ropes course" is an ideal environment for a staff retreat and will help encourage team building.

CHALLENGE #2

- **Develop a strong brand identity.**
  - *Strategy: Proceed with selection of a new logo to be used consistently on all printed materials.*

  - *Strategy: Create a new practice handbook:*
    - An updated patient handbook should be created. It should be a simple blueprint showing how to access and find satisfaction as a patient at Tennessee Allergy and Asthma Center. Its goal is to ease a patient's visit by managing expectations. It should be written and designed to be patient-friendly and be distributed to all new and returning patients.
    - This simple communication tool should include at least the following:
      - Your mission statement;
      - Your hours of service;
      - Your locations;
      - How to make an appointment;
      - Specially credentialed staff;
      - Hospital affiliations;
      - Products and services;
      - Methods of payment;
      - Emergency service; and
      - Physician biographies.

  - *Strategy: Create a sales presentation kit:*
    - An information piece should be created for your non-patient audience, such as managed care and employers. The purpose of this piece is to serve as a communication tool that will be a guide to understanding allergy and asthma care and the services provided by your physicians and staff.
    - This kit should be created in such a way that it is easily updated as your practice evolves. It must look attractive and professional. It can be a pocket-folder format or in a bound-booklet format, depending on the volume of information required. It should include at least the following:
      - Your mission statement;
      - Products and services with definitions of each;
      - Your commitment to clinical trials and research;
      - A description of outpatient testing and clinics;
      - Differentiation of the Tennessee Allergy and Asthma Center;
      - Any added value you bring to the community;

- Practice guidelines and clinical protocols which have been implemented;
- Access;
- Service;
- Quality issues;
- Location;
- Commitment to community;
- Physician bios and photos;
- History of Tennessee Allergy and Asthma Center; and
- Your commitment to patient education.

- *Strategy: Review Yellow Page ad design:*
  - Tennessee Allergy and Asthma Center should be more communicative in its Yellow Page advertising. This does not require two- or four-color advertising or a full-page ad. However, you should have at a minimum an in-column ad, and all physician names should be listed under Tennessee Allergy and Asthma Center.
  - Also, review phone directories in outlying communities where Tennessee Allergy and Asthma Center has a presence and make sure they're accurate.

- *Strategy: Develop a campaign to introduce your new doctor:*
  - Compile a short doctor bio fact sheet and include all that apply:
    - Physician name;
    - Specialty and subspecialty;
    - Board certifications;
    - Fellowship training;
    - Residency;
    - Internship; and
    - College of medicine.
  - Distribute to internal staff, referring physicians, managed care plans and/or other interested parties.
  - Schedule new physician for photography session at local photo studio. Order ten five- by-seven- inch black and white photo prints for use with press releases, printed materials and other opportunities.
  - Prepare a news release using the information noted previously.
  - Distribute the news release (with the photos where appropriate) to:
    - Local newspaper;
    - Local medical society publication;
    - Local city magazine;

- Other local publications;
- New physician's alma mater publication;
- Local radio/ TV community service programs; and
- Hospital newsletters.
- Implement an ad campaign to introduce the new doctor to the community.
- Create an ad announcement.
- Place in appropriate publications, such as:
  - Local medical society publication;
  - Local hospital newsletter;
  - Local neighborhood newspapers;
  - American Lung Association local chapter newsletter; and
  - Specialty community publications.
- Prepare and distribute an announcement card. There are three ways to prepare the announcement, including:
  - Create and print a special note card and envelope announcement;
  - Create and print a postcard announcement; or
  - Imprint on existing note card.
- Distribute announcement card to your target audience, including:
  - Referring physicians;
  - Existing patients;
  - Managed care panels;
  - Managed care administrator staff; and
  - Potential new patients (purchase a mailing list for ZIP codes in your neighborhood).
- Update Yellow Page ad to add the new physician's name.
- Update all identity materials to add the new doctor's name, such as:
  - Letterhead;
  - Patient brochure;
  - Signage; and
  - Managed care panel booklet.
- Create and print Rolodex cards to be used in appropriate ways.
- Write an introductory article about the new doctor for inclusion in your next patient newsletter or for use as an office handout.
- Conduct a referring physician campaign to introduce your new doctor.
- Write and distribute a letter announcing the new doctor's arrival and credentials.
- Have the new doctor make an introductory visit to major referrers in both primary care and pediatrics.

- Conduct a managed care campaign to introduce the new doctor:
  - Write and distribute letter announcing the new doctor's arrival; and
  - Set up a meeting for the new doctor with the medical director and provider relations' liaison.
- Conduct an open house to introduce the new doctor to the community at large (optional).
- Prepare and place a feature article related to the new doctor (if appropriate) highlighting special skills or techniques of interest to the general public (optional).

- *Strategy: Develop a system for direct mailing to current and potential patients:*
  - All Tennessee Allergy and Asthma Center patients should be maintained in a computer database so you can communicate with them as necessary. This database must be updated monthly to add new patients and delete deceased and exited patients. Communication opportunities include:
    - New products or services, such as allergy and asthma support groups or clinical trials;
    - New information about Tennessee Allergy and Asthma Center such as having extended evening and weekend hours and new locations;
    - Educational forums;
    - Patient newsletter;
    - Open house in celebration of a special anniversary;
    - Announcement of the significant community donation; and
    - New physician in the practice.

- *Strategy: Select promotional items:*
  - Order Tennessee Allergy and Asthma Center promotional items
  - Conduct an internal assessment to determine past promotional items that have been used and whether each continues to be a popular item. In addition, ask selected staff to make recommendations concerning both patient promotional items and physician and corporate promotional items.
  - Items that are appreciated by patients include:
    - Branded tissue holders;
    - Jar grippers;
    - Mugs;
    - Sport thermoses; and
    - Fanny packs.

- Items appreciated by referring physicians include:
  - Collapsible gym bags;
  - Visors;
  - Logo golf balls;
  - Appointment/date books; and
  - Electronic organizers.
- It's a good idea to work with local vendors so they benefit from your business. Some of these items can be purchased at discount stores such as Costco, Sam's or business supply houses. The patient items should have your logo on them. The physician gifts need not.
- Distribute promotional items to patients as appropriate, such as:
  - In "goody bags" when you sponsor a community event;
  - At open houses;
  - When you speak to a community group;
  - At health care expos; and
  - When you have corporate guests visit the practice.

- *Strategy: Produce and distribute a newsletter twice a year:*
  - Work with a pharmaceutical company to share the cost with your practice. Price distribution as an insert in the local newspaper. Mail to:
    - Existing patients;
    - Major employers;
    - Referring physicians;
    - Local businesses in your community;
    - Clergy in your neighborhood; and
    - Managed care administration and medical directors.

- *Strategy: Conduct a multi-media ad campaign:*
  - Create and place a series of coordinated print ads, using your logo and other identity elements consistently with the friendly theme (work with a local public relations firm to determine the optimum ad schedule). Themes should include your overall theme and your commitment to the area, your physicians ("Meet our doctors") or important information about various allergy and asthma therapies.
  - Look for opportunities to co-sponsor community events that involve print promotion.
  - Consider sponsoring the pollen report on radio. Work with a local public relations agency to determine details and feasibility.
  - Produce six 30-second television spots and run the campaign on local cable stations.

- Purchase a 13-week radio campaign. You can either have your spots produced or you can use a radio talent or some other talent who is familiar with your practice to offer testimonial or real-life experience about how your practice has helped them
- Develop six to twelve allergy- or asthma-related articles. You can create a series on a specific topic that would run regularly, such as women and allergies, children and asthma, allergy trends, current asthma care, etc. You can work with a local community paper to place the articles or you may buy space to place the articles.

- *Strategy: Take advantage of all potential speaking opportunities:*
  - Develop an allergy/asthma care talk and coordinate speaking opportunities through the hospitals, the Chamber of Commerce, and local Coalition. Target audiences include:
    - Women's groups;
    - Men's groups;
    - Senior groups;
    - Parents of pediatric allergy or asthma patients;
    - Support groups for asthma victims;
    - Animal lovers;
    - Employee organizations;
    - YMCA;
    - American Lung Association; and
    - PTA.

- *Strategy: Create media interest in your innovative approach to care:*
  - Work with a local PR agency to develop positive media relations;
  - Develop interactive win-win relations with the hospital public relations departments and suggest media opportunities to them. Based on your long-term relationships, you may want to suggest they work closely with local media to raise the level of awareness of the outpatient approach to chronic asthma therapies.

- *Strategy: Offer articles for small local publications:*
  - Hire a local writer with media placement experience to interview your physicians and specially credentialed staff about what they do as they provide allergy and asthma services in the outpatient arena. Then review your patient base for interesting human-interest stories. It is the writer's responsibility to figure out the "hook" for the paper. Most small town papers will accept articles from a writer if he/she uses a local angle and local patient.

- Write articles for the Saturday feature of the local paper. Work with your local PR agency to place the article. It will be helpful to find out the schedule of topics for that section.

CHALLENGE #3

- **Maintain and protect managed care relationships.**
  - *Strategy: Position your practice to respond to the needs of managed care:*
    - Identify the quality assurance features you have in place and itemize the tracking you use to verify their validity;
    - Document your quality of care and explain how you communicate it to managed care; and
    - Describe your internal utilization review mechanisms and why they are valid.

  - *Strategy: Position to offer exclusive contracts to managed care:*
    - Determine how to ask for and complete a request for proposal; and
    - Decide what else you must do to offer exclusivity.

  - *Strategy: Establish a variety of reimbursement mechanisms to assist your managed care partners.*

  - *Strategy: Establish risk mechanisms to assist your managed care partners.*

  - *Strategy: Educate yourself and your staff about managed care:*
    - Make sure everyone has a working knowledge of the types, operational practices, products, etc., of the area's managed care organizations. Make sure everyone understands managed care product lines, such as Medicare, Medicaid and Workers' Comp; and
    - Encourage the billing office to develop relations with an appropriate contact person at each of the managed care companies with which you do business.

  - *Strategy: Itemize your differentiation factors and "value-added" positioning as they apply to working with managed care.*

  - *Strategy: Prepare your practice to respond to managed care changes that may benefit your practice:*
    - Stay continuously aware of what is going on with the managed care organizations with which you have relationships;
    - Keep up to date on current service area expansions, additional product lines, reimbursement preferences and interest in exclusive or preferred arrangements;

- Have a solution ready to propose if a managed care organization decides to expand into additional counties or product lines;
- Decide what you will do if any of the networks you have targeted are closed to adding additional allergy and asthma providers; and
- Know your perceived position with a managed care organization before you meet in a relationship building meeting.

- *Strategy: Be prepared to generate a Request for Proposal with the following information:*
  - Copy of DEA license;
  - Copy of Tennessee license;
  - Evidence of Board Certification;
  - Copy of Professional Liability Coverage;
  - Typed summaries of malpractice claims;
  - List of hospital/facilities with which your doctors have privileges;
  - Lists of other managed care organizations with which you have contracts;
  - Current financial statement;
  - Description and location of all community offices;
  - Description of specialists and subspecialists;
  - An overall description of your operational capabilities;
  - A staffing overview, sufficient office staff training programs and specialized equipment; and
  - Your unique features, such as report time, accountability parameters, computer support and tracking mechanisms.

- *Strategy: Make sure you have materials ready that will receive the closest attention from managed care organizations, such as:*
  - How you practice allergy and asthma care efficiently through utilization tracking and outcome studies you are willing to share; and
  - The credentialing process you use to recruit new physicians.

- *Strategy: Create and maintain a database of managed care contacts:*
  - Include administrators, medical directors, physician's liaison representatives, sales representatives and marketing representatives.

- *Strategy: Develop a plan for contracting with managed care:*
  - Begin preliminary discussions with key insurers;
  - Inquire about their allergy and asthma needs;
  - Open discussions on various reimbursement models, including capitation;

- Share what differentiates you from all other allergy and asthma practices; and
- Inquire if a Request for Proposal is being distributed.

- *Strategy: Research the National Asthma and Allergy System:*
  - Determine if they are in your market area; and
  - Determine if there are benefits to developing a relationship with them.

- *Strategy: Follow up to be sure the Tennessee Allergy and Asthma Center is listed in the managed care directories:*
  - These are usually updated twice a year. It is your responsibility to be sure your listing is correct and as you want it. If you aren't listed, you will not have an opportunity to build top-of-mind awareness and brand equity.
  - As you join new panels, send a letter to appropriate referral doctors to let them know that you have been admitted to the panel and can see their referrals. It is important to communicate, as the new provider panel books are printed only periodically.

- *Strategy: Create a program for inviting managed care contacts to the practice:*
  - Invite your contacts to visit the practice and stay for lunch. Always schedule a relationship-building physician to attend the lunch.

- *Strategy: Develop a method for tracking your utilization of resources.*

- *Strategy: Develop clinical guidelines for appropriate defined care and its benefit to patients:*
  - Commit these guidelines to writing; and
  - Define your "system" of use for applying to the practice.

- *Strategy: Be prepared to communicate how your practice has invested in patient education with the goal to increase patient compliance:*
  - Create a list of patient education tools you have created and include representative samples.

- *Strategy: Conduct an annual survey of managed care plans to determine how well you are doing in regard to access, service and quality.*

CHALLENGE #4

- **Establish and maintain a strong referral physician program.**
  - *Strategy: Develop and implement a plan for physician-to-physician interactions:*
    - Tennessee Allergy and Asthma Center physicians must commit to being actively involved;
    - Tennessee Allergy and Asthma Center doctors must determine what responsibility they will take to make calls to key influencing referring physicians;
    - Create and maintain a database of referring physicians, which will include:
      - List of your top referring physicians;
      - List of primary care physicians and pediatricians on mutual managed care panels;
      - List of PCPs and pediatricians on the hospital's medical staff rosters; and
      - Lists of physicians can be purchased from the Department of Professional Regulations in your state.

  - *Strategy: Create a database of all primary care, internal medicine specialists, pediatricians, pulmonologists and other physicians with a potential to refer:*
    - Provide them with allergy and asthma updates;
    - Make an effort to entertain them in some capacity;
    - Develop a brown bag "lunch and learn" program for referring physician staffs; and
    - Offer to conduct a joint seminar to benefit their patients with asthma and allergy problems.

  - *Strategy: Develop a plan to contact new physicians in town and other potential referring physicians:*
    - Welcome them with a call or letter;
    - Add new physicians to your database; and
    - Offer to be of service and help to the newcomers as they integrate into the health care community.

  - *Strategy: Develop appropriate communication tools:*
    - Physician newsletter with case studies, new equipment, trends in treatment, etc.;
    - Reprints of published research of interest to referring physicians; and
    - Products and services fact sheet.

- *Strategy: Create effective strategies to track and continuously communicate with referrers:*
  - Create a monthly report that tracks referrals by source;
  - Create a monthly report that shows who is referring to whom;
  - Create a 90-day report to look at referral trends; and
  - Create a response mechanism if referrals appear to be slowing down or drying up.

- *Strategy: Conduct and follow up on an annual physician survey to find out how well your practice is meeting the needs of referring physicians and their patients.*

CHALLENGE #5

- **Build brand equity within the business community.**
  - *Strategy: Join the local business Coalition:*
    - Develop an interactive relationship with a liaison staff person;
    - Set up a formal meeting to learn more and to explore how providers can integrate into the Coalition;
    - Become familiar with the Coalition's long- and short-term goals;
    - Volunteer to collaborate on an allergy or asthma research project;
    - Evaluate the opportunity to underwrite or sponsor a Coalition program; and
    - Volunteer for a committee.

  - *Strategy: Create a database of Coalition Board members.*

  - *Strategy: Volunteer to work with the Coalition on outcome measurements on the treatment and management of asthma.*

  - *Strategy: Create a database of key influencers at major employers, including:*
    - CEO;
    - Human resources;
    - Benefits manager;
    - Industrial nurses; and
    - Company physicians.

  - *Strategy: Offer to provide four articles a year addressing allergy or asthma trends or treatments for their company newsletter.*

  - *Strategy: Volunteer to be a participant at their company health fair.*

CHALLENGE #6

- **Enhance patient relations.**
  - *Strategy: Create and distribute the following patient education fact sheets:*
    - What asthma is;
    - Medications for the prevention and relief of asthma attacks;
    - Bronchodilators;
    - Anti-allergic mediator agents (cromolyn);
    - Anti-inflammatory agents (corticosteroids);
    - How to use your inhaler;
    - Care of the asthmatic child;
    - How asthma is diagnosed;
    - Asthma self-care to avoid or decrease asthma episodes;
    - Asthma and exercise guidelines to lessen or prevent asthma attacks;
    - Managing allergies and asthma at school;
    - How to respond to an allergic reaction;
    - How to use metered dose inhalers and peak flow meters; and
    - The importance of sticking to treatment regimens.

  - *Strategy: Conduct an annual patient survey.*

  - *Strategy: Sponsor allergy and asthma support groups.*

  - *Strategy: Create a web page for your practice:*
    - Update it and add to it on a regular basis;
    - Support patients who use the Internet chat rooms as a support group; and
    - On a weekly basis, answer the "most frequently asked questions."

IMPLEMENTATION SCHEDULE

PHASE 1 (projects which should be initiated in the first six months)

CHALLENGE #1
- Strengthen internal relations;
- Review all print materials;
- Create a mission statement and display it throughout your Center;
- Brainstorm with your staff to determine your "value-added" advantages;
- Conduct an in-service education program to begin educating your staff about health care changes; and
- Conduct an annual strategic planning retreat.

CHALLENGE #2
- Develop a strong brand name identity newsletter;
- Create a patient handbook (incorporate your mission statement and theme);
- Review Yellow Page ad(s) and update where necessary;
- Conduct a campaign to introduce your new physician;
- Develop ongoing patient communications plan;
- Develop three patient-based talks and position to be a speaker at community meetings. Work with the hospital PR department and the wellness areas of major employers;
- Improve media relations; and
- Hire local freelance writer to write and place articles.

CHALLENGE #3
- Develop program to maintain and protect desired managed care relationships;
- Make preparations to communicate internal quality assurance programs;
- Identify who (inside the practice) will be responsible to respond to Requests for Proposal;
- Conduct an internal audit of your relations with managed care to know your patient mix;
- Review your patient mix and financials to determine your ability to capitate;
- Create your differentiation list;
- Engage in an environmental assessment to evaluate expansion or networking opportunities so as to be able to offer exclusivity;
- Initiate relationship building with multiple members of the managed care administrative teams; and
- Conduct an annual managed care survey.

CHALLENGE #4
- Establish and maintain a strong referral physician program;
- Develop a plan for physician-to-physician communication;
- Develop a plan to initiate referral physician "brown bag" lunch-and-learn programs;
- Implement referral-tracking system;
- Begin developing a program to promote allergy and asthma leadership; and
- Conduct an annual referral survey.

CHALLENGE #5
- Build brand equity within the business community; and
- Add the business community database to your mailing list.

CHALLENGE #6
- Enhance patient relations;
- Prepare and distribute patient education fact sheets;
- Create a practice Website;
- Conduct a patient survey; and
- Sponsor allergy and asthma support group.

PHASE II (projects which should be initiated in the second six months)

CHALLENGE #2
- Develop a strong brand name identity;
- Create a corporate presentation booklet;
- Continue ongoing patient communications plan;
- Order and distribute promotional items;
- Produce and distribute semi-annual newsletter; and
- Develop and implement multimedia campaign.

CHALLENGE #3
- Develop program to maintain and protect managed care relationships;
- Begin "lunch and tour" program;
- Continue discussions with key insurers; and
- Distribute corporate communication booklet to managed care.

CHALLENGE #4
- Establish and maintain strong referral physician program;
- Develop plan to meet or have contact with referrers; and
- Develop plan to communicate with new doctors entering the community.

CHALLENGE #5
- Build brand equity within the business community;
- Continue lunch-and-learn program;
- Participate in employer health fairs; and
- Distribute corporate communication booklet.

BUDGET
- Staff Retreat: $500;
- Patient handbook:
- Creation: $1000; and
- Printing: $TDB based on volume.
- Corporate booklet:
  - Creation: $2500; and

- Printing: $TBD based on volume.
- Campaign to introduce new doctor:
  - Ad creation: $ 250;
  - Ad placement: $TBD by publication selection;
  - Postcard creation: $250;
  - Distribution: $TBD by fields by zip code selection and field selections; and
  - Postage: $Bulk third-class rate.
- Fact sheet:
  - Creation: $50; and
  - Imprinting: $ 0.05 each.
- Press release :
  - Creation: $150; and
  - Distribution: $ 0.33 each.
- Mailing to referral doctors $ 0.50/piece plus postage.
- Promotion:
  - Patient giveaways $ 2.50 to $5 with a minimum of 500 pieces; and
  - Physician promotional items: $10 to $15 with a minimum of 100.
- Newsletter:
  - Creation: $1500; and
  - Distribution: TBD—will go by mail house at bulk rate.
- Allergy print ads:
  - Creation: $250 (1/4 page ad); and
  - Placement: TBD by publication selection and run.
- Lunch-and-learn programs:
  - Work with Olive Garden or other local restaurant to provide meals.

Marketing Plan of Action Example 2: Orthopaedic Practice

Strategic Marketing Plan of Action
for the
Jewett Orthopaedic Clinic

(Campaign to promote the Jewett Joint Replacement Center)

Background

For the past few years, the Jewett Orthopaedic Clinic has dedicated a large portion of its marketing budget and efforts to the promotion of sports medicine. Maximizing its position of strength and leadership as team physicians for the NBA Magic, WNBA Miracle, UCF, Rollins, IHL Solar Bears and the World Cup — through use of the theme "Your Team Physicians" — has earned excellent rewards in increased brand name identity for the Clinic.

Over the same time period, several designated subspecialty "Centers" have been identified and promoted through use of special logos, fact sheets, brochures, newsletters and other promotional activities. These include the Jewett Orthopaedic Foot and Ankle Center, the Jewett Sports Medicine Center, the Jewett Spine Center and, of course, the Jewett Hand Center. However, the area of joint replacements has not yet been highlighted in this manner.

At this time, however, the decision has been made to establish the Jewett Joint Replacement Center and to develop and implement a strategic plan of action to promote it to referring physicians, patients and other important target audiences throughout central Florida.

Marketing Goals
- Create a distinctive, yet coordinated visual (graphic) identity for the Jewett Joint Replacement Center and use it on all communications for the Center.
- Build brand loyalty for the Jewett Joint Replacement Center and be recognized as the #1 center for joint replacement care in Central Florida.
- Reinforce a favorable image of the Jewett Joint Replacement Center with all target audiences.

- Educate patients about joint replacement surgery and foster good patient relations for the Jewett Joint Replacement Center.
- Communicate success stories, new procedures and other stories of interest that would help position the Jewett Joint Replacement Center as #1.
- Inform referring physicians and managed care about the Jewett Joint Replacement Center and its services.

Target Markets

The following audiences are appropriate to be targeted for marketing efforts in a four-county central Florida area (Orange, Seminole, Lake and Osceola counties):

- **Consumers:**
  - General senior community;
  - Retirement communities; and
  - Golf communities.
- **Sports Participants:**
  - Baby boomers involved in sports.
- **Referring Physicians**
- **Managed Care Companies**
- **Other Targets:**
  - Senior organizations;
  - Senior publications;
  - Bookstores;
  - Radio programs that appeal to seniors; and
  - General media.

Marketing Strategies
Strategy #1

Build and maintain a strong brand name identity for the Jewett Joint Replacement Center with consumers in the central Florida community.

Strategy :
- Conduct a six-month saturated, yet cost-effective ad campaign promoting the Jewett Joint Replacement Center, which includes:
  - Print advertising:
    - Create and place ads in senior and specialized publications.

Figure 10-a

Jewett Joint Replacement Center Ads

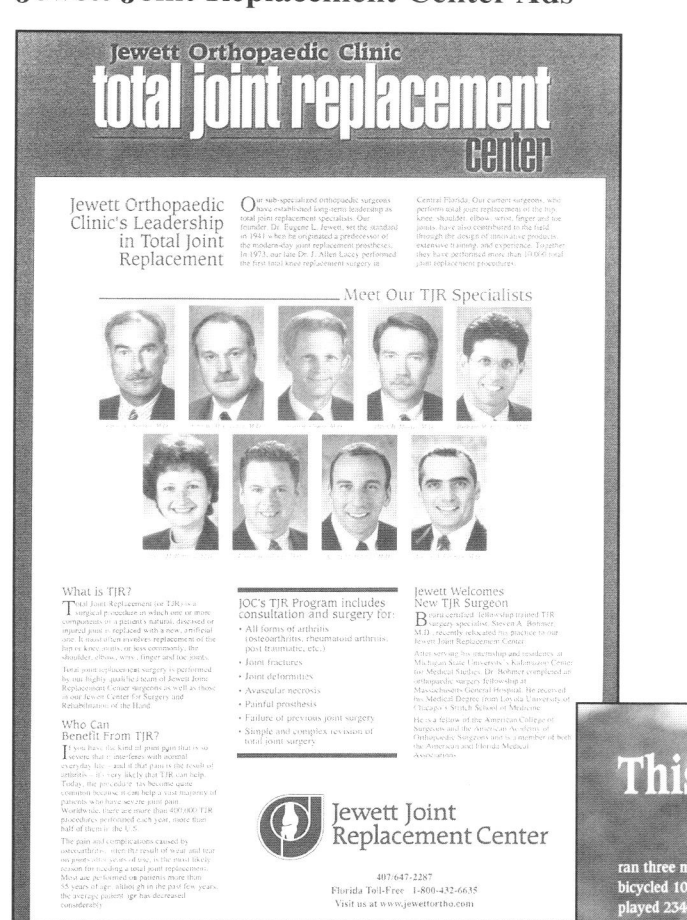

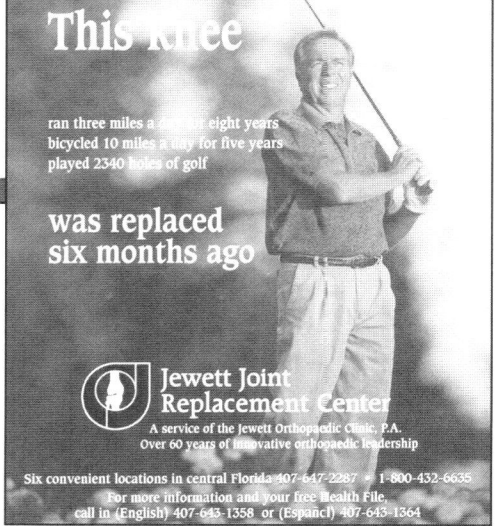

- Radio advertising:
  - Create and place 30- or 60-second spots on appropriate stations; and
  - Hire well-known former TV anchor, Ben Acrigg, to serve as spokesman — "And now, here's Ben Acrigg with the Jewett Joint Replacement Center News."

Strategy:
- Conduct a six-month public relations campaign to support the radio and print schedules. This may include planning and coordination of some or all of the following elements:
  - Media relations:
    - Utilize May, as National Health Education Month, Senior Citizens Month and Older Americans Month, to initiate an education program to both print and broadcast media;
    - Create and place articles about joint replacement care in senior publications throughout central Florida;
    - Place previously prepared articles about Jewett Joint Replacement Center doctors in local newspapers in surrounding counties;
    - Write and distribute appropriate news releases (new procedures, updates);
    - Set up and coordinate broadcast interviews;
    - Pitch patient profile and success stories, such as "Now Mable can go back to the bowling team," "Harry is back on the golf course," etc. ; and
    - Explore other feature story ideas, such as "1000th knee replacement patient," unusual patients, helping a needy patient, etc.

  - Community relations:
    - Create and deliver community talks about joint replacement care at:
      - Nonprofit organizations;
      - Retired military;
      - Radio talk shows (new procedures, updates);
      - Local clubs; and
      - Local bookstores.

  - Patient relations:
    - Refine previously designed total joint replacement sub-logo to identify the Jewett Joint Replacement Center within the Jewett Orthopaedic Clinic. Use consistently on all appropriate materials, such as fact sheet and brochure;

Figure 10-b
Jewett Orthapaedic Clinic

- Develop appropriate communication tools, such as:
  - Jewett Joint Replacement Center patient information brochure; and
  - Jewett Joint Replacement Center fact sheet shell and imprinted fact sheets.
- Sponsor or participate in special events, such as:
  - Health fairs;
  - AARP retirement meetings;
  - Senior expos;
  - Morning coffee/tour of facility (food draws people!); and
  - Special promotions, in conjunction with radio stations or senior publications.
- Produce and distribute special "Health File" for patients.

Figure 10-c

Sample Health File

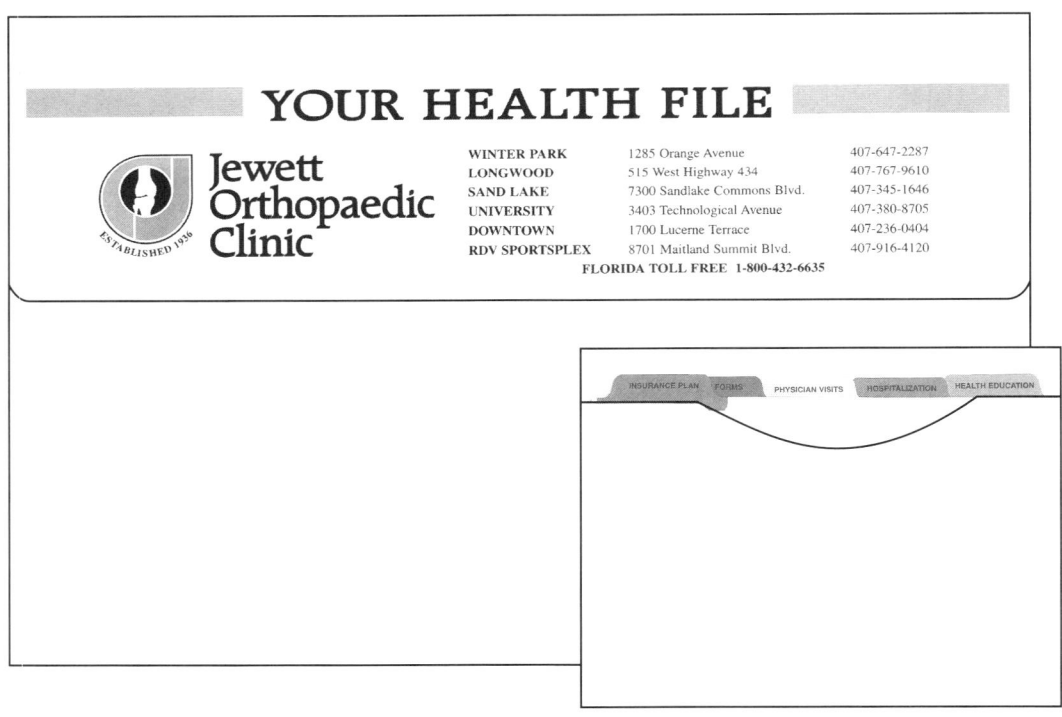

Strategy:
• Review Yellow Page ads to include the Jewett Joint Replacement Center .

Strategy #2

Provide excellent patient education about joint replacement care and foster patient satisfaction for the Jewett Joint Replacement Center.

Strategy:
• Distribute brochure and fact sheets as follows:
    • Give to all existing patients at all six offices (as they arrive for appointments);
    • Give to all new patients and other interested parties;
    • Provide supply to the nine joint replacement doctors for handouts as appropriate; and
    • Hand out at trade shows and other events.

Strategy:
• Conduct a semi-annual patient satisfaction survey of Jewett Joint Replacement Center patients.

Strategy:
• Sponsor joint replacement support group.

Strategy #3

Inform referring physicians about the newly identified Jewett Joint Replacement Center.

Strategy:
• Identify selected key influencers and meet with them to explain the mission and goals of the Jewett Joint Replacement Center.

Strategy:
• Conduct direct mail letter campaign to inform all appropriate referral physicians about the Jewett Joint Replacement Center.

Strategy:
• Conduct a referral physician survey focusing on the Jewett Joint Replacement Center.

Strategy:
- Create and distribute twice-a-year doctor-to-doctor letter or fact sheet with updated information and trends on joint replacement care.

Strategy:
- Invite selected referring physicians to be guests at Magic, Miracle and/or Solar Bears games.

Strategy #4

Inform selected managed care partners about the newly identified Jewett Joint Replacement Center.

Strategy:
- Conduct direct mail letter campaign to inform selected managed care directors about the Jewett Joint Replacement Center.

Strategy:
- Invite selected managed care directors to tour the Jewett Joint Replacement Center.

Implementation

We recommend beginning implementation of this campaign in May to coincide with special national events and continuing through October. To achieve this schedule, we will begin immediately to research media, begin production of collateral materials, and create ads and radio spots. An implementation schedule is attached.

Budget

Budget for a campaign similar to this will fall into a wide range, depending upon the costs of your specific market. To be effective, we recommend at least a six-month campaign, so sufficient budget should be allocated to cover that time period. In addition to media placement costs, be sure to include cost of producing one or more radio commercials.

Marketing Plan of Action Example 3: Breast Care Practice

Strategic Marketing Plan
for the Breast Care Center

(Campaign to achieve brand equity)

Background

The Breast Care Center is a new, subspecialized practice formed by two female physicians, a surgeon and a radiologist, to meet the breast care needs of Central Florida women. It is the only female two-specialty partnership in Orlando, offering both diagnostic testing and breast surgery in one practice. This team approach gives patients the convenience of comprehensive on-site evaluation of breast problems — including state-of-the-art diagnostic imaging equipment, surgical consultative services and sophisticated follow-up — in a "caring, compassionate" atmosphere.

Breast care is the sole passion of this practice, which is dedicated solely to the evaluation, diagnosis and treatment of breast disease. These two physicians have commitment to provide high-quality clinical breast care, as well as to provide the sensitivity and emotional support that many women need. They believe it's *the right way* to provide breast care — because it means patients can achieve the best possible outcomes.

In addition to efficient, effective, nurturing care, the goal of the Breast Care Center is to provide "one-stop shopping" for women. This practice believes that women should not have to wait one to three weeks to get answers after finding a lump in a breast or having an abnormal mammogram. Therefore, they have designed a system where women don't have to wait — results are provided in two to three days or even sooner.

Overview

This Strategic Marketing Plan outlines the marketing recommendations that we believe are necessary to position the Breast Care Center to begin to achieve "The Dream" as it has been described to us through conversations and our brainstorming questionnaire. Combining your input and our knowledge, experience and expertise, we have analyzed the threats and opportunities in the current environment as well as your specific strengths and weaknesses.

Our recommendations are designed to help you maximize the advantages the Breast Care Center has to offer, based on today's health care situation as it exists in the central Florida marketplace. It should be noted that no in-depth market research has been conducted to determine specific demographics and market potential. Also, this plan includes only those initial strategies that could be considered Phase 1 of your marketing plan. Obviously, marketing cannot simply stop after this initial phase. It is an ongoing process that must be viewed as an investment in your practice. We will, therefore, review this plan after six to nine months to determine direction from there.

Situation Analysis

Because the Breast Care Center is a new practice, and we have conducted limited research, the situation analysis will be, of course, fairly brief. A list of perceived strengths, weaknesses, threats and opportunities as well as other pertinent information has already been compiled from your responses to our questionnaire. A copy is included with this report.

A list of current possible Breast Care Center competitors is also attached, including general surgeons, OB/GYNs, imaging centers, etc.

Because managed care is an extremely vital part of any health care practice today, we have included a special section outlining the state of managed care in central Florida as well as general ideas concerning how physicians must position to attract and maintain managed care contracts. This section follows the Situation Analysis.

Our previously discussed Referring Physician Program presents a background on the importance of referral relations in today's health care environment, along with methods of fostering these positive relations. A copy of it is also attached with this plan.

Managed Care

As you recognize, managed care plans have become a customer in line with referring physicians and patients. They are the initial hurdle that has to be cleared to access patients in a managed care setting. Being excluded from the network excludes the group or practice from seeing patients represented by the managed care plan.

The lesson learned from saturated managed care markets is that relationships are key. Once managed care plans have good relationships with providers, they try to maintain those relations. It is, therefore, imperative that the Breast Care Center develops relationships with the managed care plans that are deemed most appropriate and desired.

There are three areas within a managed care organization that are key to ongoing, productive relationships with a group practice. These are:
- Utilization management;
- Provider relations; and
- Member service/satisfaction.

In addition, it is very important for the group practice administrator to develop and maintain productive working relationships with two key influencers within the managed care organization. These are the health plan administrator and the medical director. This is important because these are the people who make the decisions.

These decisions include expansion of the plan and its panel, who they are going to contract with, who they are going to terminate and whom they want to be more cooperative with in negotiating sessions.

What do managed care plans want in their relationships? The criteria listed, via the personal interview process, include:
- Price;
- Cost-effective behavior;
- Quality of care;
- Geographic coverage;
- Privileges at participating hospitals;
- Philosophic accord;
- Willingness to work collaboratively to develop organized systems of care with other appropriate physicians;
- Understanding of how the managed care plan does business and why they do it that way;
- Long-term partnerships with physicians;
- Practice differentiation and value; and
- Physicians who score high in outcome measurements using MedisGroup data.

Once you enter into a contractual relationship, you have to work at developing the relationship. You need to become interactive with the medical director, upper-level administration and your provider relations representative. You need to talk with them and position the Breast Care Center to assist them with their needs. You need to ask the questions, "How can we best help you reach your goals concerning breast care?" and "What role would you like us to play?" This is attitudinally opposite from the traditional physician disposition of "This is what we do, and we're great at it. Managed care should be grateful to work with us."

It will be very productive for the Breast Care Center to share its cost-reduction strategies with managed care partners, both current and future. You need to volunteer to participate in and even lead meetings with your managed care partners and fellow referring physicians on Organized Systems of Care. Organized Systems of Care will be a collaborative approach of typically connected primary care physicians and specialists who will approach treatment plans to disease that provide the appropriate outcome while reducing waste and duplication between physicians and various ancillary services.

Your goal is to become the provider resource in breast care to all your managed care partners. This must be initiated by your on-going interactive relations with the medical director or local plan contact. It requires phone calls, letters and personal visits.

Throughout the Breast Care Center's initiatives to service managed care partners, you are in a time period in which it is to your advantage to be proactively responsive to their needs.   During negotiations and discussions have ready at your finger tips:
- An accurate and current physician roster;
- Current addresses of your physicians and any satellite offices;
- All collateral material necessary for contracting such as:
  - Copy of DEA license;
  - Copy of Florida license;
  - Evidence of Board Certification;
  - Copy of Professional liability fact sheet; and
  - Typed summaries of any malpractice claims.
- List of hospitals and outpatient centers BCC has privileges with, including the type of privileges; and
- Utilization management data from the hospital's MedisGroup records.

How to position for risk

The shift to physician capitation in the future creates a need for the Breast Care Center to focus on considering whether it can position itself to take risk through capitated arrangements. Payers are looking for cost-effective physicians.

Getting experience with prepaid contracts is crucial to future survival. The focus on managing risk begins with running an efficient practice and cutting all unnecessary administrative costs to the bone. As a practice, you must be able to maintain quality, employee morale and patient service within the budget managed care plans are willing to pay.

The bottom line for managed care is: **BE EASY TO WORK WITH AND RESPONSIVE TO THEIR NEEDS.**

Marketing Goal

To achieve #1 "brand equity" in breast care imaging and surgery in Central Florida.

Marketing Positioning

What can make the Breast Care Center unique in the eyes of potential target markets?

1. Convenient location.
2. A practice which emphasizes patient care, quality and sensitivity.
3. An innovative place to go for breast care diagnosis, screening, imaging and treatment due to the unusual partnership of female, board certified surgeon and radiologist.
4. A place to go where each patient is treated as a priceless commodity.
5. A practice whose doctors regularly perform a high volume of specialized procedures with good outcomes.
6. A place to go for privacy and surgical excellence.

Research and Planning

1. Identify computer software.
2. Identify appropriate community sponsorships.
3. Identify advertising media sources and cost:
   - Print;
   - Radio;
   - Billboard; and
   - Other.
4. Identify radio talk show opportunities.
5. Identify potential networking opportunities for the physicians.
6. Develop a list of managed care administration contact people.
7. Review Yellow Page opportunities.
8. Identify promotional item and cost.
9. Identify referring practices to invite to staff wine and cheese parties.

10. Identify areas in the business community in which to become involved.
11. Identify sponsorship opportunities in areas pertinent to women's issues.
12. Update physician bios.
13. Update physician photos.

Marketing Challenges
1. Develop a strong brand name identity:
   • Internal
2. Develop a strong brand name identity:
   • External
3. Develop a program to maintain and protect desired managed care relations.
4. Build and maintain a strong referral physician program.

Challenge #1

Develop a strong brand name identity:
   • Internal strategies

   Strategy #1: Create print materials to help develop a consistent image:
   • Work with the physicians to design the Breast Care Center logo;
   • Create letterhead package which will include:
      • Standard letterhead;
      • # 10 envelope;
      • Second sheets;
      • Note card;
      • Note card envelope;
      • Business cards (3);
      • Appointment card;
      • Rolodex card;
      • Fact sheet shell;
      • Note pad; and
      • Mailing label.
   • Edit patient information fact sheets on various topics.

   Strategy #2: Create a mission statement:
   • Use the mission statement on practice brochure, presentation kit and in reception area and patient rooms. This should be created by the practice, not marketing.
   Strategy #3: Develop a practice handbook:
   • Distribute to all new and returning patients; and
   • Distribute at community talks.

Figure 10-d

Breast Care Center brochure

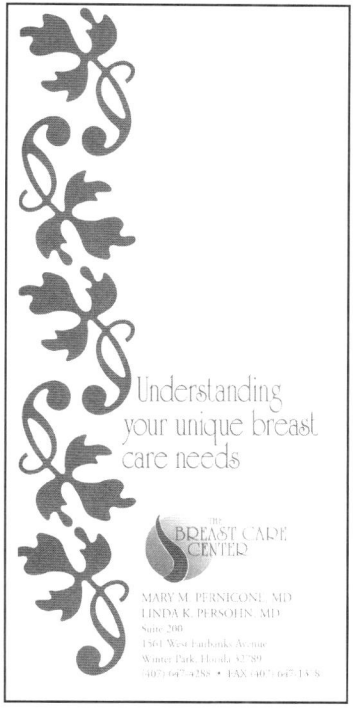

Strategy #4: Develop a coordinated system for direct mailings to potential patient base on various topics, including:
- Information about the Breast Care Center and its mission and services;
- Announcement of new facility;
- Educational forums/seminars; and
- New products and services.

Strategy #5: Select a promotional item for give-a-way purposes:
- Custom bag with logo containing candy; and
- Present as each patient exits the practice after a visit.

Challenge #2

Develop a strong brand name identity:
- External strategies

Strategy #1: Develop a program to integrate the Breast Care Center into the community:
- Join appropriate Chambers of Commerce and underwrite programs of special interest to women:
  - Greater Orlando Chamber of Commerce; and
  - Winter Park Chamber of Commerce;
- Join the Central Florida Health Care Coalition;
- Develop corporate sponsorships;
- Join and underwrite programs of the Women's Resource Center;
- Join and provide sponsorship for Sexual Assault Resource Center; and
- Utilize appropriate communication tools.

Strategy #2: Develop and plan a multi-media ad campaign:

Figure 10-e

Breast Care Center Ads

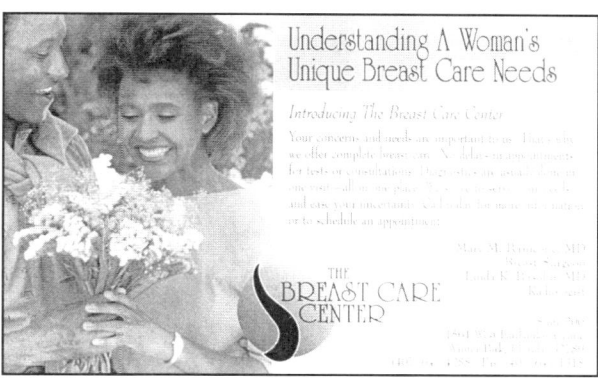
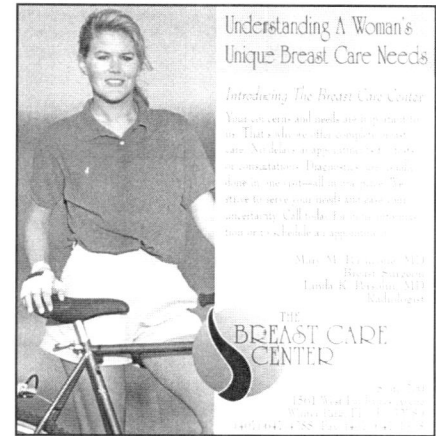

- Produce print ads:
  - Produce and place print ads;
  - Create 4-color ad;
  - Create black and white ads, including shell;
- Produce and place a radio campaign:
  - Create 30-second spots;
- Produce and distribute a direct mail announcement card for opening:
  - Create and print post card;
  - Purchase list.

Strategy #3: Review and standardize Yellow Page ad design.

Strategy #4: Take advantage of speaking opportunities:
- Women's groups;
- Teen programs; and
- American Cancer Society.

Strategy #5: Sponsor and become actively involved in an appropriate community project.

Strategy #6: Create media interest in your innovative approach to care:
- Develop relations with reporters through lunches or phone conversations; and

- Send news releases when there is value for the community at large to be informed via a print story.

Strategy # 7: Promote new technology, which appeals to target markets:
- Create and distribute a press release on Sentinel Node Mapping; and
- Invite the media to see application of the technology, if appropriate.

Strategy #8: Write article(s) for small local publications.

Challenge # 3

Develop a program to maintain and protect desired managed care relations.

Strategy # 1: Create and maintain a current database of managed care contacts and communicate with them as appropriate:
- When the contract is signed, make sure you are included on the available provider list. Follow up to be certain you are not inadvertently excluded when the panel brochure is reprinted;
- When you are added to a panel, send a letter stating you are now a plan participant able to see their referrals for breast mammography/surgery and a Breast Care Center brochure to all potential referring physicians on the panel; and
- Develop a relationship with the director of utilization review.

Strategy #2: Create a program for inviting managed care contacts to the practice:
- Engage in personal contact twice a year (one can be a phone call and one should be a personal visit).

Strategy #3: Create a database (or at least a list) of primary care, internal medicine and OB/GYN physicians who participate in plans on which you want to maintain relations:
- Communicate by letter or post card that you are on the plan and available to see their patients for cost-effective, quality, satisfactory patient care;
- Research what is important to them;
- Provide them with news of interest;
- Develop a positive interactive relationship with them; and
- Entertain them.

Strategy #4: Develop a game plan for contracting with managed care.

Strategy #5: Determine the "value-added" or Breast Care Center differentiation factor:
- Commit this list of factors to writing; and
- Be prepared to discuss these when you have personal visits with managed care contacts.

Strategy #6: Develop a method for tracking utilization of resources in your outpatient setting.

Strategy #7: Request and know your MedisGroup status from the hospital for inpatient care.

Strategy #8: Communicate to managed care how your practice has invested in patient education.

Strategy #9: Develop collateral materials that will position the Breast Care Center as having developed a cost-effective "System Approach to Breast Care."

Challenge #4

Build and maintain a strong referral physician program.

Given the current and expected future environment, BCC's primary marketing challenge is to establish and maintain positive referring physician relations. Current and potential referring physicians must be identified, understood, courted and treated as team members.

Strategy #1: Create a referral database that can be easily accessed and used to mail merge communications from BCC.

Strategy #2: Create effective strategies to track and continuously communicate with referrers:
- Create a monthly report that tracks referrals by source;
- Create a monthly report that shows who is referring to whom;
- Create a 90-day report to look at referral trends; and
- Create a response mechanism if referrals appear to be slowing or drying up.

Strategy #3: Develop and implement a plan for physician-to-physician interactions:
- BCC doctors must commit to being actively involved;
- BCC doctors must determine what responsibility they will take to

make one-on-one calls to referring physicians and potential referring physicians;

- Determine the number of calls or visits to be made each week by each BCC doctor;
- Determine who will create the list of primary care and internal medicine doctors and OB/GYNs to be contacted and what the focus of the interaction will be. Who will create the referral physician call sheet to eliminate duplicate calls? Currently available:
  - List of top referring physicians known to doctors by historical experiences;
  - List of primary care, internal medicine and OB/GYN physicians on various BCC managed care panels;
  - List of all physicians who share presence on various community managed care panels;
  - List of physicians from hospital rosters;
  - List of physicians in current medical society membership in all three counties;
  - List of physicians which can be purchased from the DPR; and
  - Call upon as many of them personally as possible to outline the BCC commitment.

Strategy #4: Develop appropriate communication tools, including:
- Initial press release announcing the opening of BCC;
- Rolodex card/business card;
- Pre-printed referral pads with maps;
- Fax referral form for inter-office use;
- Letter of commitment of quality of care;
- Procedural guidelines and practice parameters;
- Physician-to-physician handbook;
- Physician newsletter with case studies, new equipment, trends in treatment;
- Reprints of published research; and
- Case studies of unusual interest.

Strategy #5: Develop a mechanism to summarize any doctor-to-doctor contacts that focus on dissatisfaction or super satisfaction in working with the BCC:
- These should be jotted on notes and turned in for summarizing, working on solutions and re-communicating with the referring physician.

Strategy #6: Develop a plan to contact new physicians in town or other potential referring physicians:
- Immediately call or write a letter of welcome and introduction;
- 30 days later, follow up with:
  - BCC brochure;
  - Rolodex card;
  - Managed care panel participation;
  - Appointment pads with map; and
  - BCC brochure and newsletter or case study.

Strategy #7: Commit to a referring physician protocol :
- Determine phone call return time;
- Determine patient referral access time;
- Commit to report time turn-around;
- Develop quality of care protocols;
- Create and distribute procedure fact sheets;
- Involve referring doctors in treatment plans; and
- Distribute physician newsletter or case studies.

Strategy #8: Develop a campaign to meet all female referring physicians:
- Invite all female referring physicians for a screening mammogram and work up during May (Mother's Day) or another selected month.

Strategy #9: Develop a campaign to meet all OB/GYN physicians:
- Develop ongoing breakfast, lunch or office visit meetings for referral physicians to get feedback on what they expect from your group;
- Create a referral physician outreach program;
- Identify any existing problems;
  - Change perceptions; and
  - Respond to needs.
- When a BCC physician receives a complimentary letter from a patient, copy the letter and send it to the referring physician with a note that says, "Thought you might like to see that your patient had a positive experience in our office";
- Develop lunch-and learn programs for referring physician office staffs;
- Schedule "wine and cheese" after hours for office staff of referring ;practices; and
- Offer to do a joint seminar to their patients which involves both specialties.

Strategy # 10: Develop a campaign to meet all FP physicians and other potential referrers:
- When a BCC physician refers a patient back to a primary care physician or surgeon for basic care, send a letter to that primary care physician to let her know the referral was made; and
- See previous suggestions for OB/GYN.

Strategy #11: Enhance BCC's image in the medical community by emphasizing leadership, education and training:
- Prepare and distribute fact sheets; and
- Conduct in-service education programs.

Marketing Plan of Action Example 4: Primary Care Practice

Marketing Plan of Action
for
Primary Care Specialists

(Campaign to introduce new doctor and new office)

GOAL

To create a community-based primary care practice for Dr. Parvis Brahman and to announce the opening of a new Primary Care Specialists (PCS) office in Longwood and the immediate surrounding area. PCS is a small practice management group that employs 20 physicians in this region. After recently opening a new office, the practice initiated this campaign to introduce that office and a new physician to the community.

Challenge
To develop top-of-mind awareness for Dr. Brahman and the new office within the Longwood and the immediate surrounding community.

Targets
- Community physicians;
- Patients;

- Key community influencers; and
- Community at large.

Objectives
- To build overall brand name identity for Dr. Brahman;
- To announce the new office and to build overall awareness of its location in Longwood; and
- To provide patient education and foster patient satisfaction.

Research and Planning
- Identify list(s) of potential patients and key influencers in the community surrounding the new office ;
- Identify all potential referral sources in surrounding community; and
- Identify appropriate media for news release(s), ad campaign and /or media stories.

Positioning
- Capitalize on the location of the practice in Longwood; and
- Capitalize on Dr. Brahman's background (education/tra ning and past experience).

MARKETING STRATEGIES
- Write and distribute news release announcing Dr. Brahman's appointment and opening of office in Longwood (with photo).

- Create and place an announcement ad introducing Dr. Brahman and announcing the location of the new PCS Longwood office. Emphasize new patients and walk-ins welcome. Place in appropriate media, such as:
  - Central Florida Family;
  - Central Florida Physician;
  - Local community paper(s) for Longwood, Sweetwater, Springs areas; and
  - Area retirement center newsletters.

- Prepare and use distinctive identity materials (using logo) of the new office, such as:
  - Stationery, appointment card, business card, Rolodex card, etc.;
  - Patient handbook;
  - Signage; and
  - Map showing office location.

- Determine what differentiates this practice from others in the area, such as special hours, special services, special expertise, service orientation, walk-in acceptance, etc. Emphasize this "added value" in all public relations and advertising materials.

- Create a direct mail list of potential patients in the surrounding community ($30,000 household income residents in Longwood and immediate surrounding area zip codes).

- Create an attention-getting oversized direct mail postcard using practice logo and Dr. Brahman's photo announcing new office location (include map). Distribute to above list.

Figure 10-f

Sample Direct Mail Flyer

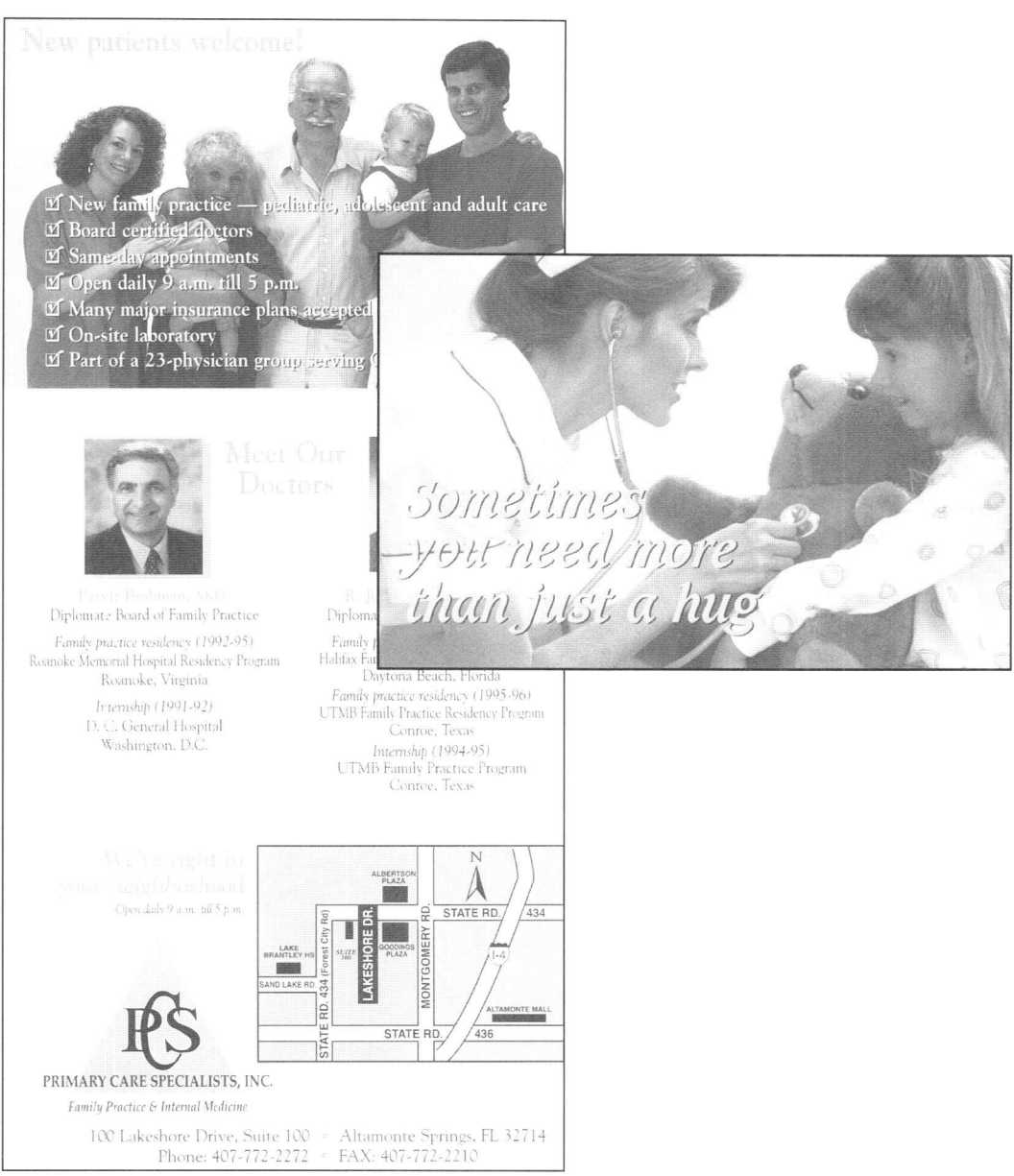

- Write a letter and mail to existing PCS patients announcing the new location and inviting them to remain with the practice at the new location.

- Create a direct mail list of potential referrers in the surrounding area, such as:
  - Area physicians in such specialties as obstetrics/gynecology, orthopaedics, cardiology, dermatology, plastic surgery, dentistry, orthodontics, etc.;
  - Merchants;
  - Restaurant managers;
  - School principals;
  - PTA presidents;
  - Mayor;
  - Police and fire department managers;
  - Emergency services managers;
  - Post office manager;
  - Holistic providers (complementary and alternative), such as nutritionists, therapists, salons, spas, massage therapists and skin care specialists;
  - Pharmaceutical and lab reps; and
  - Managers of retirement centers, nursing homes and skilled living facilities.

- Write announcement letter(s) with appropriate message(s) and mail with Rolodex card to list of potential referrers in area.

- Dr. Brahman or Office Manager should make personal visits to other physicians, key community influencers and other potential referrers (see list).

- Investigate Welcome Wagon services and participate if available in Longwood area.

- Schedule patients "creatively" (such as all within the same two-hour period) to make the practice look busy (until it gets busy).

- Update Yellow Pages to add Dr. Brahman's name.

- Create and print bio sheet for Dr. Brahman for distribution to patients (use photo).

- Provide printed patient education fact sheets.

- Create a "Welcome to our practice" poster with Dr. Brahman's photo and bio and place on an easel in the reception area. Leave it in place for 90 days.

- Conduct a patient satisfaction survey after office has been open nine months.

- Track patients to help measure practice growth.

- Create a new office fact sheet and distribute (hand out or mail) to patients, referring physicians and/or other interested parties. Information should include the following:
  - New location;
  - Address;
  - Map;
  - Phone number;
  - Fax number;
  - Managed care plans;
  - Hours of operation;
  - Services;
  - Special staff;
  - Special equipment; and
  - Special procedures or technologies.

- Create an attractive, informative patient handbook (by end of year) including the previously noted information plus other appropriate information. Distribute in office and mail to new patients prior to their visits.

- Purchase a customized promotional item and personally (Office Manager) distribute to first 500 patients as well as key community neighbors. Suggestions include a Band-Aid holder, first-aid kit, first-aid chart or other useful household item related to health care.

- Sponsor soccer or Pop Warner team for fall.

- Join Longwood Chamber of Commerce.

- Write articles about practical health care topics and offer to senior centers for use in their newsletters.

- Volunteer to participate in career day at local schools.

- Make a small ($200) contribution to the local school for purchase of medical supplies so principal's budget can be used for other things.

- Offer special programs, such as flu shots in the fall. Promote through ads and direct mail to targeted groups as appropriate.

Marketing Plan of Action Example 5: Neurosurgical Practice

Orlando Neurosurgical Associates

(1996 Strategic Marketing Plan of Action to Establish Leadership in Radiosurgery)

Situation Analysis/Background

Stereotactic radiosurgery is a major new outpatient surgery technique which supplements currently accepted treatments for selected brain tumors and arterovenous malformations (AVMs). This procedure, which controls tumor growth, is bloodless — requiring no surgical incision to expose the tumor. It is performed by a multidisciplinary team of neurosurgeons, radiation oncologists, medical physicists, radiologists, nurses, computer specialists and technicians, who unite to provide comprehensive care before, during and after the procedure.

The long-term effect of radiosurgery, as well as its prolonged effectiveness, is still unknown. For example, it has not yet been shown that this technique lengthens the survival rate of patients with malignant tumors over conventional therapy. Therefore, caution must be exercised when this alternative therapy is recommended to patients over a well-established medical or surgical therapy. However, if predictions hold true, this breakthrough in neurosurgery and radiation therapy may very well become the treatment of choice for many neurological diseases in the future.

Currently, there are two types of equipment that can be used to perform radiosurgery — the Gamma Knife, which utilizes cobalt radiation, and the X Knife, which uses x-ray beams.

Although they are both new here, the Gamma Knife has been around since the late 1960s and is well-known outside the U.S. The X Knife was pioneered in the 1980s at the Brigham and Women's Hospital and Joint Center for Radiation Therapy, Harvard Medical School. The Gamma Knife costs about $3 million, while the X Knife, which operates in combination with a linear accelerator, costs only about $400,000.

Both the Gamma Knife and the X Knife are (or will soon be) available in the central Florida area — Orlando Regional Healthcare System (through MD Anderson Cancer Center) has the X Knife, and Florida Hospital has the Gamma Knife.

A type of radiosurgery, which is performed using the X Knife, has emerged as the new hope for difficult brain lesions adjacent to crucial brain structures. This procedure, called fractionated stereotactic radiation therapy, delivers radiation in several stages, allowing normal brain tissue to recover from the injurious effect of the radiation while controlling the growth of tumor cells. This is the preferred radiosurgery technique for most pediatric tumors and tumors that infiltrate the brain tissue, which are the most common brain tumors in adults.

According to the producers of the Gamma Knife, it is considered by some to be especially useful when conventional surgical techniques pose high risks, such as in the presence of other illnesses or when a patient's age prohibits standard surgery.

More than 6,000 brain tumor patients have been treated with the Gamma Knife at five sites worldwide, with no procedure-related mortality. Another 2,000 or so patients with AVM have undergone Gamma Knife radiosurgery. Between 80 and 87 percent of AVMs were completely obliterated and 11 percent are partially obliterated within two years. No standard surgical therapy has achieved such a favorable outcome with such a low rate of morbidity.

At this time, Orlando Neurosurgical Associates' Dr. PSL and Dr. LR are the only two neurosurgeons in central Florida who are trained to perform radiosurgery using either the X Knife or the Gamma Knife.

Dr. PSL has agreed to become involved in the Florida Hospital radiosurgery program with the Gamma Knife. Dr. LR would like to be recognized as having strong involvement in the MD Anderson Cancer Center program with the X Knife. It is believed that Orlando Neurosurgical Associates will be able to reap the most benefit in this manner, as they can cover each other's patients and be responsive to insurance plans and both hospital systems.

Hospital Marketing of Radiosurgery

ORHS/MD Anderson Cancer Center

Dr. WJ has visited one-on-one with physicians to tell them about radiosurgery. A large mailing was sent to all physicians who refer to MD Anderson Cancer Center physicians, and a large mailing also was sent to educate managed care providers about the subject. Case reviewers and care coordinators were invited to a full day at MD Anderson for a multidisciplinary program, involving everything the Center does, including telemedicine contacts with Houston headquarters. Radiosurgery was probably included, but it was not highlighted. There has been no emphasis on radiosurgery mailings to physicians who would refer to neurosurgeons, only to cancer referring physicians.

One or two media articles have appeared concerning radiosurgery, and Barbara West of Channel 9 TV taped a story. However, to date, it has not aired.

For 1996, ORHS/MD Anderson plans to produce a physician newsletter highlighting radiosurgery and the X Knife, which will be distributed to 16,000 physicians throughout Florida. The focus will be on neuro-oncology. They also plan to focus on radiosurgery at special luncheons with managed care representatives.

Dr. WJ is working to create the Brain Tumor Center, which he expects to be funded by ORHS/MD Anderson Cancer Center. He will appoint members to act in leadership roles and to participate in the treatment of patients. However, patients are rarely referred directly to the radiation oncologist from the referring physician. They are usually referred to the neurosurgeon, who then refers them to MD Anderson as necessary.

He believes the Brain Tumor Center will be of value for the following reasons:
1. A proven history in multidisciplinary care;
2. Strengths of MD Anderson;
3. An extensive array of clinical protocols;
4. The first center to perform radiosurgery and brain tumor seed implants;
5. The only FDA-approved fractionated stereotactic system with over 40 procedures already performed;
6. Purchase of an intraoperative optical tracking system for optimal removal of brain tumors;
7. Member of the Brain Tumor Cooperative Group and active participant in NCI trials through the Radiation Therapy Oncology Group; and
8. Active quality of life studies for brain tumor patients.

Dr. WJ has expressed an interest in having Dr. PSL and Dr. LR serve as joint medical directors of the Brain Tumor Center. It seems like it would be a marketing benefit to position Dr. LR and Dr. WJ together where possible to show a team approach to case management. The same can probably be done with Dr. PSL.

Florida Hospital

Florida Hospital has a formidable marketing machine, and its plan to market the Gamma Knife is extensive. It is targeting 12 counties throughout central Florida. It plans to work with hospitals through the hospitals' tumor boards. Those talks, which are over one hour and meet CME requirements, will offer CME credits as an incentive for referring physicians. Some talks will only be 10 minutes and will be at the invitation of the hospitals in these 12 counties. Response to date has been positive.

Currently, Dr. S, Dr. L, Dr. A, Dr. PSL and Dr. LR will be given equal opportunity to sign on to a comprehensive calendar schedule as designated expert speakers.

Florida Hospital has purchased a marketing package offered by the Gamma Knife producers. Basically, the marketing plan has been adjusted to involve:

- A "dog and pony show" at outlying hospitals;
- A mailing to physicians in 12 counties, which will include letters, fact sheets and brochures. The brochures will include photos and bios of those neurosurgeons practicing radiosurgery at Florida Hospital;
- A mailing to managed care insurance panels;
- A meeting with insurance case managers; and
- An address on the Internet listed under both Florida Hospital and Gamma Knife.

It has been made clear that Florida Hospital has strong sensitivities to make all marketing opportunities available to all neurosurgeons who are credentialed to perform radiosurgery with the Gamma Knife. However, it will be the responsibility of the neurosurgeons to be actively involved in Florida Hospital's marketing efforts. If commitments are made to marketing and then not honored by the neurosurgeons, it will be highly frowned upon, and eventually, there will be consequences.

We recommend that Dr. PSL and Dr. LR work very hard to remain active at the Florida Hospital Gamma Knife Center as well as ORHS/MD Anderson Cancer Center.

The marketing efforts of ORHS/MD Anderson and Florida Hospital will help to position the individual Orlando Neurosurgical Associates physicians as leaders in radiosurgery. However, Orlando Neurosurgical Associates has a responsibility to shore up efforts to be leaders and educators and sensitive consultants to referring physicians.

The challenge becomes to align with the marketing efforts of both ORHS/MD Anderson and Florida Hospital and utilize these opportunities along with marketing strategies created and implemented by Orlando Neurosurgical Associates. Altogether, these multiple efforts will create a foundation of radiosurgery leadership for Orlando Neurosurgical Associates physicians.

Strategic Marketing Plan of Action

GOALS

We have identified the following goals for the marketing plan of action:
- To establish Orlando Neurosurgical Associates as the leading providers of stereotactic radiosurgery in the central Florida area; and
- To identify Orlando Neurosurgical Associates as leaders in both the X Knife and Gamma Knife procedures for radiosurgery.

STRATEGIES (CHALLENGES)

We have identified the following strategies (which we call challenges) to achieve Orlando Neurosurgical Associates' goals:
- Establish and maintain a strong referral physician program designed to obtain radiosurgery referrals;
- Develop a strong brand name identity in radiosurgery;
- Strengthen internal relations to prepare for a leadership presence in radiosurgery;
- Develop programs to enhance managed care's knowledge of Orlando Neurosurgical Associates' leadership in radiosurgery;
- Maximize on Orlando Neurosurgical Associates' membership in the Central Florida Health Care Coalition; and
- Identify and develop radiosurgery media opportunities.

CHALLENGE #1

- *Establish and maintain a strong referral physician program designed to obtain radiosurgery referrals.*

  Note: Given the current and expected future environment, this is Orlando Neurosurgical Associates' primary marketing challenge. Current and potential referring physicians must be identified, understood, courted and treated as team members at a higher than ever level.

  Strategy: Create a database of all family practice physicians, internal medicine specialists, pediatricians, OB/GYNs, neurologists, endocrinologists, ophthalmologists, ER doctors, ENT doctors, radiologists, neurosurgeons who are not accredited to use the X Knife or Gamma Knife, and other physicians with the potential to refer for radiosurgery:
  - Keep in mind that there is a "need to know" about radiosurgery, even among physicians who are involved in the patient care chain but are not direct referral sources. This database should be stored in

your office on a PC which also has the capacity to mail/merge and to access the Internet;

- Use this database to educate physicians about radiosurgery and communicate Orlando Neurosurgical Associates' radiosurgery involvement (see following):
  - Lists to be considered:
    - List of referring physicians known to Orlando Neurosurgical Associates practice;
    - List of referral physicians with whom Orlando Neurosurgical Associates shares various managed care panels;
    - List of all physicians who refer to MD Anderson Cancer Center;
    - List of all physicians who refer to WDW Cancer Center;
    - List of physicians from both hospitals' rosters; and
    - List of physicians which can be purchased from the DPR.

Strategy: Develop and distribute appropriate communication tools, such as:
- 1996 update letter on state of the art and the Orlando Neurosurgical Associates involvement in 40 radiosurgery procedures;
- Letter of commitment to quality care;
- Physician newsletter with radiosurgery case studies, new equipment, trends in treatment, etc.;
- Reprints of published research;
- One-page radiosurgery case study with photos and CT scans (twice a year); and
- Other case studies of unusual interest.

Strategy: Create and distribute a referral physician survey with a special segment on radiosurgery services:
- Conduct survey annually.

Strategy: Create a six- to eight-minute videotape using Orlando Neurosurgical Associates surgeons to educate about radiosurgery:
- Use the Radionics tape as a model; and
- Distribute to all referring physicians.

Strategy: Offer to review patient x-rays if the referring physician has questions about whether or not a patient is a candidate for radiosurgery:
- Distribute letter to all referring physicians to let them know this.

Strategy: On the day of the visit by a patient for whom you recommend radiosurgery, fax a short note with your report to let the referring physician know your findings:
- Include a notation that a full written report will follow by mail; and
- You gain advantage by doing the unexpected, but valued, behavior by communicating with a referring physician on the same day. The goal is to get their attention, serve their patients and please both referring physicians and patients in order to increase your referral base. Whatever you do toward this end definitely will be beneficial over time.

Strategy: Develop and implement a plan for physician-to-physician interactions regarding radiosurgery:
- Orlando Neurosurgical Associates doctors must commit to being actively involved;
- Determine what responsibilities each will take to make one-on-one calls to referring physicians and potential referring physicians;
  - Determine focus of the interaction — try to make it a combination of personal calls in conjunction with mailed communication.

Strategy: Create effective strategies to track and continuously communicate with radiosurgery referrers, including:
- Monthly report that tracks referrals by source;
- Monthly report that shows who is referring to whom;
- Quarterly report to look at referral trends; and
- Response mechanism if referrals appear to be slowing or drying up.

Strategy: Enhance Orlando Neurosurgical Associates' image by emphasizing leadership, education and training in radiosurgery:
- Prepare and distribute fact sheets; and
- Conduct in-service education programs.

Strategy: Position to speak frequently about radiosurgery at grand rounds and other rounds:
- Distribute letter to hospitals.

Strategy: Commit to a referring physician protocol for radiosurgery:
- Determine phone call return time;
- Determine patient referral access time;
- Commit to report time turn-around;

- Develop quality of care protocols;
- Create and distribute radiosurgery procedure fact sheets ;
- Involve referring doctors in treatment plans; and
- Distribute physician newsletter or case studies on radiosurgery.

Strategy: Develop a campaign to meet all physicians who have the potential to refer radiosurgery:

- Develop ongoing breakfast, lunch, office or phone meetings for referral physicians to educate them about how radiosurgery benefits particular brain tumor problems;
- Create a referral physician outreach program:
  - Identify any existing problems;
  - Change perceptions; and
  - Respond to needs.
- When an Orlando Neurosurgical Associates physician receives a complimentary letter from a patient, copy the letter and send it to the referring physician with a note that says, "Thought you might like to see that your patient had a positive experience in our office"; and
- Work cooperatively with both hospitals to develop lunch-and-learn programs for referring physician office staffs to educate them about radiosurgery.

Strategy: Develop a plan to contact new physicians in town or other potential referring physicians to educate them about radiosurgery:

- Immediately call or write a letter of welcome and introduction;
- Give personal attention when possible. Invite them out for a breakfast or lunch meal/meeting to learn about them and to share Orlando Neurosurgical Associates' radiosurgery experience. Include your other services, products and access for new patients;
- Seven to 10 days later, follow up with:
  - Orlando Neurosurgical Associates radiosurgery referral physician brochure;
  - Rolodex card;
  - Managed care panel participation;
  - Appointment pads with map; and
  - Orlando Neurosurgical Associates brochure and newsletter or case study.
- Add all new physicians to your existing referral database; and
- Make a commitment to be a responsible communicator to the referring physician.

Strategy: Eliminate commercials from a half-hour radiosurgery television special *(see Challenge #2)*:
- Distribute to all referring physicians.

CHALLENGE #2
- *Develop a strong brand name identity in radiosurgery.*

Strategy: Create a logo and tagline to be printed on special Orlando Neurosurgical Associates stationery to position your practice as leaders in radiosurgery:
- Make sure that all radiosurgery print materials have a consistent corporate identity;

Figure 10-g
Orlando Neurosurgical Associates

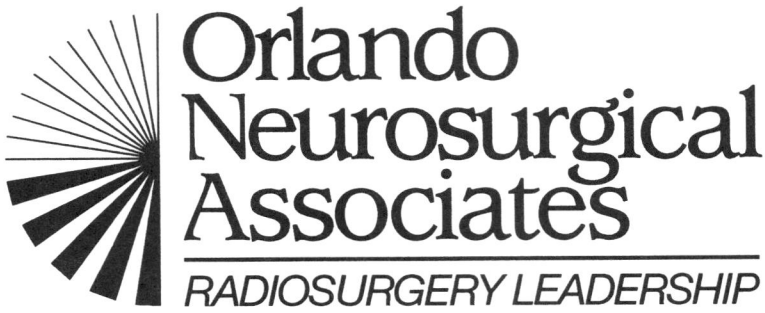

- Use only these materials for all radiosurgery communication; and
- Create and/or transfer appropriate information on to special radiosurgery fact sheet shells.

Strategy: Create a new physician referral brochure on radiosurgery, including both the X Knife and the Gamma knife and both hospital systems:
- It should be a simple blueprint showing how to access and understand the treatment planning of patients who are candidates

for radiosurgery at Orlando Neurosurgical Associates' practice. The goal is to ease a referral visit at Orlando Neurosurgical Associates by managing expectations. The brochure should be written and designed to be friendly and be distributed to all existing and potential referring physicians;

- This simple communication tool should include:
  - Your mission statement;
  - Your "value-added" positioning;
  - Your location;
  - Radiosurgery training and experience of neurosurgeons;
  - Hospital affiliations;
  - Products and services, in addition to radiosurgery leadership; and
  - Physician bios.

Strategy: Discuss with ORHS/MD Anderson and Dr. WJ the possibility of having ORHS/MD Anderson Cancer Center create and place print ad(s) on the Brain Tumor Center and the X Knife:

- Feature Dr. LR with Dr. WJ in the ad.

Strategy: Develop a mechanism for routine communication with ORHS/MD Anderson and Florida Hospital Gamma Knife Center. *Building community relations with multiple collaborative partners is one of the big secrets and keys to surviving the turmoil of the next three years:*

- Participate in MD Anderson newsletter twice a year;
- DB at MD Anderson will be using the quarterly newsletter and half-day seminars to increase awareness of radiosurgery. Dr. WJ will be creating the Brain Tumor Center as a center without walls in MD Anderson. Make recommendations, participate and follow through to benefit from mutual marketing opportunities. Orlando Neurosurgical Associates should take advantage of the partnership with MD Anderson and ORHS by having routine dialogue with the hospital system. You will benefit from their research and knowledge and be better able to plan strategies for marketing your practice. By aligning closely with their outreach efforts, the Orlando Neurosurgical Associates brand equity will be enhanced; and
- MAB, Florida Hospital, will have multiple opportunities to position Orlando Neurosurgical Associates physicians in the marketing efforts for the Gamma Knife. Again, if Orlando Neurosurgical Associates continues to participate and remains hospital-friendly, your brand name identity as leadership in radiosurgery will be enhanced.

Strategy: Produce and purchase air time for a 30-minute television news special on trends in neurosurgery, cooperatively with both hospital systems, to increase awareness of radiosurgery.

Strategy: Create and distribute a radiosurgery T-shirt to increase overall awareness of radiosurgery:
- Offer to patients when they have radiosurgery treatment; and
- Distribute in other appropriate ways.

Strategy: Place ads in *Orlando Magazine, Central Florida Physician and Hospital News.*

Strategy: Review Yellow Page ad design:
- Add radiosurgery, Gamma knife and X Knife capabilities.

CHALLENGE #3

- *Strengthen internal relations to prepare for a leadership presence in radiosurgery.*

Strategy: Working as a practice, which involves clinical, business and staff leadership, determine what differentiates Orlando Neurosurgical Associates from all competitors as it applies to leadership in radiosurgery:
- Develop a list of valued attributes that will be useful to your future allied partners and customers;
- Prioritize until you have three to five strong points of differentiation;.
- Commit this list to writing; and
- Define what is valuable and why this differentiation is important to those you will be partnering with or recipients of neurosurgery/radiosurgery services.

Strategy: Educate staff about radiosurgery procedures:
- Plan a series of in-service educational meetings for Orlando Neurosurgical Associates staff; and
- Inform and involve staff in understanding the clinical aspects and patient services which your practice provides to the radiosurgery patients from the local or outreach communities. This can at times be a point of conversation when communicating with referral staff offices. Involving the staff enables them to communicate more empathetically with patients, to become more sophisticated ambassadors for Orlando Neurosurgical Associates and to be more knowledgeable about case management when radiosurgery is the treatment of choice.

Strategy: Establish internal marketing person as the vital link between Orlando Neurosurgical Associates and both hospitals:
- Doctors should set up meeting with each hospital and introduce internal marketing person as their trusted delegate.

CHALLENGE #4

- *Develop programs to enhance managed care's knowledge of Orlando Neurosurgical Associates' leadership in radiosurgery.*

Strategy : Create and maintain a database of managed care contacts:
- Include the administrators, medical directors and provider relations liaison or utilization managers.

Strategy: Create an open-door policy with both MD Anderson Cancer Center and Florida Hospital so they will feel free to invite you to attend (as available) when they offer lunch-and-learn programs on radiosurgery to managed care contacts:
- Provide your newly created referral physician brochure on radiosurgery to the guests in attendance via the host organization; and
- Communicate Orlando Neurosurgical Associates' investment in patient education, enhanced service and increased patient satisfaction.

Strategy: Create a database of primary care, internal medicine, pediatrics, endocrinologist, neurologists, general neurosurgeons and OB/GYN physicians on plans in which Orlando Neurosurgical Associates participates:
- Provide them with radiosurgery and neurosurgery news of interest to them; and
- Entertain them.

Strategy: Develop a game plan for quarterly communication with managed care:
- Share with them what differentiates you from all other neurosurgeons providing radiosurgery expertise; and
- Inquire if there is a Request for Proposal being developed to carve out radiosurgery procedures. (If so, respond appropriately.)

Strategy: Conduct an annual survey to be distributed to managed care plans to ask how well Orlando Neurosurgical Associates is doing in regard to access, service and quality.

CHALLENGE #5

- *Maximize Orlando Neurosurgical Associates' membership in the Central Florida Health Care Coalition.*

  Note: One of the key trends in health care today is the emergence of business coalitions and alliances. No matter how health care reforms itself, the business community plays a major role on a daily basis. There are about 90 coalitions in the U.S. today, and certain generalities seem to be universal to the majority of them. They have a commitment to shared values which involve both community-based reform and value-based purchasing. There are diverse approaches of employer coalitions, and each coalition is at different stages of maturity. However, it is safe to state that they come together in a community for one or more of the following reasons:
  - *Contracting for health services;*
  - *Developing and sharing information;*
  - *Improving the quality of health care services;*
  - *Educating consumers;*
  - *Improving the health of the community and;*
  - *Leading the business community in rallying to address health care issues.*

  Community-based reform means:
  - *Health care is delivered locally;*
  - *Purchasers and consumers require accountability; and*
  - *Local presence enriches local relationships and individual commitments toward them.*

  Value-based purchasing means:
  - *Given information on the price and quality of health care services, consumers and purchasers will seek to maximize their value.*

  Strategy: Create a database of key influencers at major employers:
  - Chief Executive Officers;
  - Chief Financial Officers;
  - Chief Operating Officers;
  - Human Resource Managers;

- Benefits Managers; and
- Industrial nurses.

Strategy: Include these target groups in your mailings of case studies, fact sheets and press releases.

Strategy: Create and distribute your radiosurgery referral brochure with a cover letter to members of the Coalition Board.

Strategy: Develop an interactive relationship with the administrator of the Coalition:
- Seek to do a research project collaboratively with the Coalition.

CHALLENGE #6

- *Identify and develop radiosurgery media opportunities.*

  Strategy: Explore radiosurgery media opportunities:
  - As you develop interactive win-win relations with both brain tumor centers and medical oncology public relations departments, you can suggest media opportunities. You may want to suggest they work closer with appropriate consumer and medical print media, such as *Orlando Magazine, Central Florida Physician and Hospital News,* to raise the level of awareness of the brain tumor treatment sophistication and procedures taking place within the hospitals. With patient permission, you may encourage having a media person job-shadow one of the neurosurgeons for a half day. If you do this, we recommend that it include time in the CT area as well as with the medical oncologist and physicists as they create the therapy plan. Include either breakfast or lunch with the physician and others, who are available on the radiosurgery team. A meal opportunity allows the reporter to ask good questions and feel that he/she gets a sense of the physician's neurosurgery leadership above and beyond the procedure. Prior to this event, be sure that the Orlando Neurosurgical Associate physician understands that this is a time to highlight the practice's overall leadership in neurosurgery. Everyone must benefit by sharing health care information and education.

  Strategy: Work with both hospitals to develop TV human interest news stories.

Strategy: Author articles relating to radiosurgery for small local publications:
- Hire a writer with media placement experience or agency to interview Orlando Neurosurgical Associates' physicians and other specially credentialed staff about what they do as they provide neurosurgery services in the outpatient environment. Then, review your patient base for interesting human interest stories. It is the writer's responsibility to figure out the "hook" for the paper. There are many small publications in the central Florida area that will accept articles from a writer if they use a local angle, such as a local patient; and
- Write an article for *Hospital News,* which is distributed throughout most of the state.

Implementation Schedule and Responsibilities

To assist Orlando Neurosurgical Associates in determining marketing priorities, Medical Marketing makes the following recommendations. We recognize, however, that your input is necessary to determine if these recommendations are appropriate.

Project implementation

These databases should be created immediately and maintained regularly (all the responsibility of internal ONA staff):
- Database of all referring physicians and potential referrers;
- Database of managed care companies; and
- Database of physicians with which Orlando Neurosurgical Associates shares managed care panels.

These communication tools should be created immediately (unless indicated, all can be responsibility of internal ONA marketing staff or can be outsourced):
- Radiosurgery identity materials, including custom logo, stationery and fact sheet shells;
- Radiosurgery referring physician handbook;
- Radiosurgery fax report shell;
- Radiosurgery ad or ads (should continue throughout year);
- Radiosurgery T-shirt (distribute throughout year);
- Radiosurgery fact sheets (internal ONA responsibility); and
- Yellow Page ad review (internal ONA responsibility).

These letters should be written and distributed as soon as possible (all the responsibility of internal ONA staff):
- 1996 annual update for referring physicians with offer to review x-rays;
- Letter to both hospitals with offer to speak at grand rounds, etc.; and
- Letter to managed care (continue each quarter).

These internal projects should be accomplished immediately (all the responsibility of internal ONA staff):
- Determine and commit to writing Orlando Neurosurgical Associates' "value-added" differentiation;
- Educate staff about radiosurgery; and
- Establish internal marketing person as vital link with hospitals.

During the second quarter of 1996 (March – June), the following projects should be started (these can be done by internal ONA marketing staff or outsourced):
- One-page radiosurgery case study (create and distribute);
- Six to eight minute videotape (create and distribute); and
- Media stories.

These projects should be started by the third quarter of 1996 (July – September):
- Physician newsletter featuring radiosurgery (responsibility of internal ONA marketing staff or can be outsourced); and
- Program to meet new physicians in community (responsibility of ONA doctors).

Fourth quarter (October – December) projects include:
- Referral physician survey (responsibility: can be done internally or outsourced);
- Managed care survey (responsibility: can be done internally or outsourced);
- 30-minute television special — for airing and distribution of commercial-free special to referring physicians during the first quarter of 1997 (must be outsourced);
- Data base of key influencers at major employers — also include on mailing list for case studies, fact sheets and press releases (responsibility of internal ONA staff);
- Mailing of radiosurgery referral handbook with cover letter (responsibility of internal ONA staff); and
- Development of interactive relationship with Coalition administrator (responsibility of internal ONA marketing staff and/or doctors).

On-going program implementation

In addition to these projects, there are a number of ongoing programs which should be incorporated into the normal, every day "how we conduct business" system at Orlando Neurosurgical Associates. Obviously, all these fall under the responsibility of internal staff and/or doctors.

These include the following:
- Use of fax report for all radiosurgery consults;
- Physician-to-physician interactions;
- Tracking of radiosurgery referrals;
- Commitment to referring physician protocol to radiosurgery;
- Campaign to meet all potential radiosurgery referring physicians;
- Routine communications with ORHS/MD Anderson Cancer Center and Florida Hospital;
- Open-door policy with both ORHS/MD Anderson Cancer Center and Florida Hospital;
- Quarterly communications program with managed care; and
- Exploration of media opportunities (with hospitals).

Budget

The following is a very rough estimate of costs that may be incurred for projects which should or could be outsourced. Since there are so many variables involved in most of these projects, these figures should by no means be considered firm estimates.

Communication tools:
- Radiosurgery identity materials, including custom logo, stationery and fact sheet shells — $3,000 plus printing;
- Radiosurgery referring physician handbook — $2,000 plus printing;
- Radiosurgery fax report shell (included in identity package);
- Radiosurgery ad or ads — 3 ads @ $500 each plus placement costs throughout year; and
- Radiosurgery T-shirt (distribute throughout year) — $8 to $12 each, based on quantity of 100.

Second-quarter projects:
- One-page radiosurgery case study — $500 to $1000 plus distribution;
- Six to eight minute videotape — $16,000 to $22,000 plus dups and distribution; and
- Media stories (print) — $250 to $500 each.

Third-quarter projects:

- Physician newsletter featuring radiosurgery — $2,500 to $3,000 plus printing and distribution.

Fourth-quarter projects:

- Referral physician survey — $500 plus printing and distribution;.
- Managed care survey — $500 plus printing and distribution; and
- 30-minute television special — $25,000 to $45,000

11

Marketing Resources

"I am still learning."
— Michelangelo

Never underestimate the power of the Internet

Did you know that your patients now can get an "on-line physical?" Furthermore, if their on-line doctor agrees that they need help, they will receive an on-line prescription for Viagra—and it will be filled on-line!

In mid-1999, estimates of the adult on-line community in the United States range from 59 million to as high as 110 million. According to the weekly on-line newsletter *Iconocast,* some four million Websites already are estimated to exist on the Internet, with 235,000 being added each month. Reportedly, over 40 percent of Americans have Internet access either at home or at the office, and by 2000, more than seven trillion e-mails will be send annually in the U.S.

No matter how astounding the numbers, the facts are obvious. Through this new technology, your patients now have easy access to a wide range of resources on the information superhighway—and they're using this information to educate themselves about their health and their family's health. It is imperative that you recognize the role the Internet is playing in the life of your patients. The practice that is not sensitive to this important tool loses an opportunity to relate to the empowered patient.

The Internet is used to: research all types of information about disease; to look for treatment alternatives; to find connections with strangers who are struggling with similar problems; and to communicate around the world from a computer. For better or for worse, it allows patients to educate themselves as they never before could.

It does not mean that all the information patients find on the Internet is valid. In fact, misinformation and inaccuracies abound in cyberspace. However, it does mean that when you develop your marketing plan, you must consider this communication tool, in both the areas of branding and patient relations.

Other physicians find e-mail convenient for answering simple patient questions or discussing minor patient problems. If you decide to use e-mail in this manner, however, be sure you make your policies clear on your Website and in your patient brochure or other communication materials. For example, let patients know who will read the e-mail (staff or only doctor) and when it will be answered (how quickly). You should also remind patients that e-mail is not always secure.

Figure 11-a

Internet resources

There are literally hundreds of resources patients can use to access health information these days. Some practices use fact sheets to provide search engines that are popular and easy to use. These include but are not limited to the following sites:

HotBot www.hotbot.com
This is easy to use and has powerful capabilities.

Yahoo! www.yahoo.com
This is one of the oldest and best known search engines. Yahoo is primarily a directory rather than a search engine.

AltaVista www.altavista.com
AltaVista is one of the largest search engines on the Web with 150 million Web pages in its database.

Lycos www.lycos.com
This is both a search engine and a Web directory.

Excite www.excite.com
Excite features a special search tool that looks for typed-in key words and also for ideas closely related to the words in the query.

Northern Lights www.northernlights.com

Web pages are listed by rank, relevance, subject, type, source and language

Snap www.snap.com

This is a joint venture between CNet and NBC. It aims to provide what a Website has to offer so visitors can decide it they want to visit.

Other e-mail health care site addresses (the author does not necessarily endorse these companies or products):

- National Institute of Health's Medical Library www.nlm.nih.gov
- Mayo Clinic www.Mayohealth.org
- NetWellness www.netwellness.org
- OncoLink www.cancer.med.upenn.edu
- Department of Health and Human Services www.healthfinder.gov

Marketing worksheet: 7 steps to introducing a new doctor

Figure 11-b

Sample Doctor Introduction

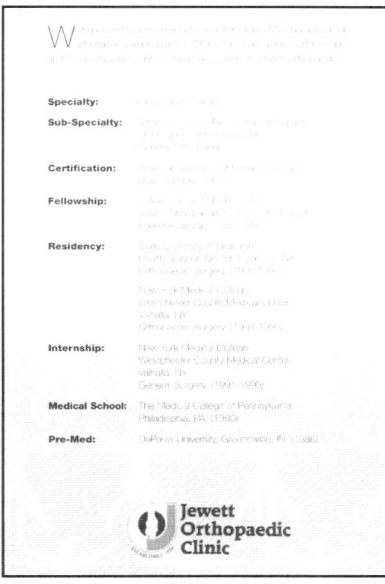

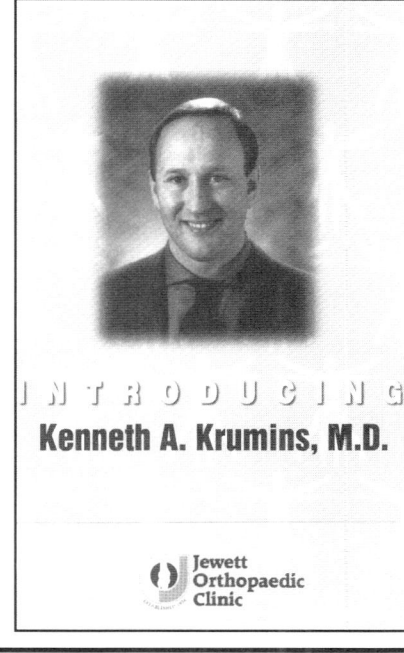

1. Prepare a physician bio — include information about your practice — logo, name, address, zip code, phone, fax, e-mail address plus physician's biography information:
    *   Specialty;
    *   Subspecialty;
    *   Board certification;
    *   Fellowship;
    *   Residency;
    *   Internship; and
    *   Medical college.

2. Prepare and distribute a press release — this introduces the new physician and provides background information, hospital affiliations and background on the group.

3. Conduct research — in preparation of compiling a media list database. Media kits can be ordered from the following prior to purchasing of ad/announcement space:
    *   Daily or weekly newspapers;
    *   Magazines or other local public publications;
    *   Medical society publication;
    *   Local radio stations;
    *   Public radio and television stations; and
    *   Special community organizations relating to the new physician's interest or expertise.

4. Create an introduction ad:
    *   Size/dimensions;
    *   Color or black and white; and
    *   Camera-ready mechanical.

5. Purchase ad space.

6. Create an announcement card — which can be a postcard or note card in an envelope. This will be distributed to:
    *   Referring physicians;
    *   Patients;
    *   Managed care companies; and
    *   Purchase lists of local residents with specific predetermined qualifications such as size of family, income, location, age and employment.

7. Remember miscellaneous details:
    *   Update all print material;
    *   Update Yellow Page ads;
    *   Hold an open house to introduce the new physician;
    *   Develop a schedule to introduce a new physician to your top 20 referring physicians; and
    *   Create a poster with the new physician's photo and credentials and place it in the reception area of all offices.

MARKETING WORKSHEET:
12 Steps to Marketing a New Medical Practice

1. Create and distribute an introductory letter:
    *   Prepare letter/introduction;
    *   Explain what the practice is;
    *   Explain how the practice works;
    *   Explain the benefits of the practice; and
    *   Include important practice information:
        *   Practice name;
        *   All locations;
        *   Phone;
        *   Fax;
        *   E-mail;
        *   Web page address; and
        *   Specialty area.

2. Develop an identity (logo):
    *   Distinctive;
    *   Memorable;
    *   Graphic;
    *   Easy use;
    *   One or two colors; and
    *   Use consistently on all communication about new product or service.

3. Prepare stationery package:
    *   Letterhead;
    *   Second sheet;

- #10 envelope;
- Note card;
- Note card envelope;
- Business cards;
- Appointment cards;
- Labels; and
- Rolodex cards.

4. Prepare patient handbook and include:
   - Welcome;
   - Address;
   - Phone number;
   - Fax number;
   - E-mail address;
   - Web page address;
   - Description of specialty if applicable;
   - Office locations and hours of operation;
   - System for calling the office and having calls return by the physician or other clinical personnel;
   - System for making appointments;
   - What to expect during the first appointment;
   - What to do during an emergency;
   - Fees, billing and insurance;
   - Hospital privileges;
   - Prescription refill policy;
   - Special staff;
   - Special services;
   - Physicians and short bios;
   - Location map; and
   - Other pertinent information.

5. Prepare and distribute a press release about opening the new office:
   - Compile a media list database (prepare in a format for mailing labels). Information should include: editor, health feature writer, address, phone, fax and e-mail address. Include:
     - Local newspaper;
     - Business newspaper;
     - Hospital newsletter;
     - Medical society publication;
     - Radio talk shows;

- • Medical health care reporters;
- • Associations of interest to the practice; and
- • Groups of interest to the practice.
- • Mail with a five-by-seven black and white photo when applicable.

6. Implement an ad campaign:
   - • Create ad;
   - • Identify all possible media where introductory ad or ads should be placed such as:
     - • Local medical society publication;
     - • Local hospital newsletters;
     - • Local neighborhood newspapers; and
     - • Specialty publications.

7. Request media kits from appropriate publications and schedule ad run.

8. Prepare and distribute announcement card:
   - • Create and imprint an announcement with or without a photo;
   - • Distribute your announcement;
   - • Identify the target audience such as referring physicians, managed care plans, potential patients; and
   - • Use a mail house when purchasing lists.

9. Place Yellow Page ads for the practice.

10. Conduct a referral physician campaign:
    - • Distribute letter/announcement; and
    - • Visit potential referrers.

11. Conduct managed care campaign:
    - • Request applications;
    - • Apply to be on the panel; and
    - • Read all contracts before signing.

12. Investigate other promotions to introduce the new practice such as:
    - • Welcome Wagon;
    - • Mailing stuffers; and
    - • Promotional items.

Conclusion

Well, there you have it. Everything you need to know about marketing your medical practice in the service-oriented environment of the new millennium. All the tools you need to get yourself—and your entire organization—off dead center and on the road to achieving your goals.

To summarize, here is my recommended 10-point plan for marketing success:

10-point marketing plan for the new millennium

1. Keep your customers coming back—by treating them like individuals.
2. Understand who your customers are—and what they want.
3. Don't forget the basics.
4. Know yourself—and your practice.
5. Empower and support your staff.
6. Retreat—to move forward strategically.
7. Recognize and respect referrers.
8. Get the most from your hospital relationships.
9. Take advantage of proven marketing techniques.
10. Emulate other successful practices.

Remember, marketing is not a sign of weakness. It is a re-investment in your practice. And, there is no deep, dark secret or magic bullet that will assure success. On the other hand, it is not as simple as some may think. Like any worthwhile activity, it takes a bit of planning, time and effort. In addition, it may require a change of attitude, and it definitely requires a commitment by everyone involved in the practice—from the very top right down to the front-line staff.

Ultimately, it comes down to keeping your customers happy. It comes down to common sense.

I urge you to use the knowledge you've gained from this book to take the action you feel is right for your practice. Apply it to your everyday life by preparing a comprehensive strategic game plan, by adopting the policies and procedures that will help guide you toward a successful future. Then, implement your plan, one customer at a time.

You have the tools. ***Now, just do it!***

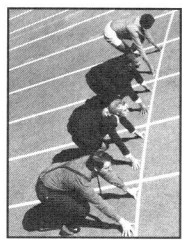

Appendix

SAMPLE MARKETING MATERIALS

The following section includes several samples that may give you ideas as you create marketing materials for your practice:

1. Fact sheet shell imprinted

2. Neurosurgery practice identity package

3. Cardiology newspaper ad

4. Dermatology practice identity package

5. Practice services brochure

6. Specialty services brochure

7. Cardiology patient newsletter

Fact sheet shell imprinted

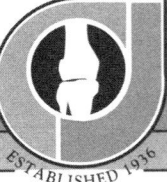

Jewett Orthopaedic Clinic

Over 60 Years of Orthopaedic Leadership

Monday through Friday 8:30 AM to 5:00 PM • Call 407-647-2287

Our phone is answered 24 hours a day • Outside the area call 1-800-432-6635
Visit us at www.jewettortho.com

What is a Physician Assistant?

(Also known as a PA)

Our PAs

Steven E. Anderson, PA-C
Chief Physician Assistant Steve Anderson received his Physician Assistant Degree and Associate of Applied Science Degree from Catawba Valley Technical College in North Carolina. He joined JOC in 1996 and has almost 20 years of experience as a PA.

Leticia Camacho-Mojica, PA-C
Physician Assistant Leticia Camacho-Mojica received a Bachelor of Science/Health Science Physician Assistant Degree at the State University of New York (SUNY) Science at Brooklyn/Downstate. She joined JOC in 1997 and has additional qualifications in both basic and advanced cardiac life support.

Jared A. Reiss, PA-C
Jared Reiss joined JOC's Physician Assistant staff in 1998. He received his Physician Assistant Degree from Kettering College of Medical Arts in Ohio, and he has additional qualifications in both basic and advanced cardiac life support.

PAs are Physician Assistants, and they have been part of the U.S. health care system since the 1960s. They are licensed or certified health professionals who provide a broad range of medical and surgical services, under the supervision of a physician.

Increasingly recognized as quality health care providers, PAs can diagnose and treat illness and injuries and often exercise a degree of autonomy in their decisions as they strive to help meet the needs of patients.

The following information will tell you more about the role of PAs in a medical or surgical practice. If you have any questions at any time, please feel free to ask us.

What does a PA do?

Physician Assistants perform physical exams, diagnose illnesses, develop and carry out treatment plans, order and interpret lab tests, suture lacerations, apply casts, assist in surgery, and provide patient education and preventive health care counseling.

To allow the PA/physician team to be efficient in extending care to patients, most states do not require PAs and their supervising physicians to be at the same location. All state laws require the supervising physician to be immediately available for consultation when the PA is seeing patients, either in person or by telephone.

How are PAs educated?

Most PA programs require applicants to have had previous health care experience and some college education. The typical

applicant has a Bachelor's Degree and more than four years of health care experience prior to joining the program. Nurses, EMTs and paramedics frequently apply to PA programs.

All PA programs are accredited by one independent organization supported by the American Medical Association, the American Academy of Family Physicians, the American College of Surgeons and other national medical organizations. Whether located at a college, university, medical school or teaching hospital, all PA programs must meet the same accreditation standards.

Accredited PA programs provide a broad education in primary care medicine in two phases. The first phase includes lectures and lab sessions in anatomy, physiology, pharmacology, microbiology and other basic sciences.

The second phase is spent in clinical rotation in such specialties as family medicine, internal medicine, pediatrics, emergency medicine, obstetrics and gynecology, geriatrics, surgery, psychology and other specialties. During this period, students diagnose and treat patients.

A PA's education doesn't stop after graduation. Like other medical professionals, PAs are committed to lifelong learning. PAs take continuing medical education classes throughout their careers and are required to take a national recertification exam every six years.

(Continued on back)

Neurosurgery practice identity package

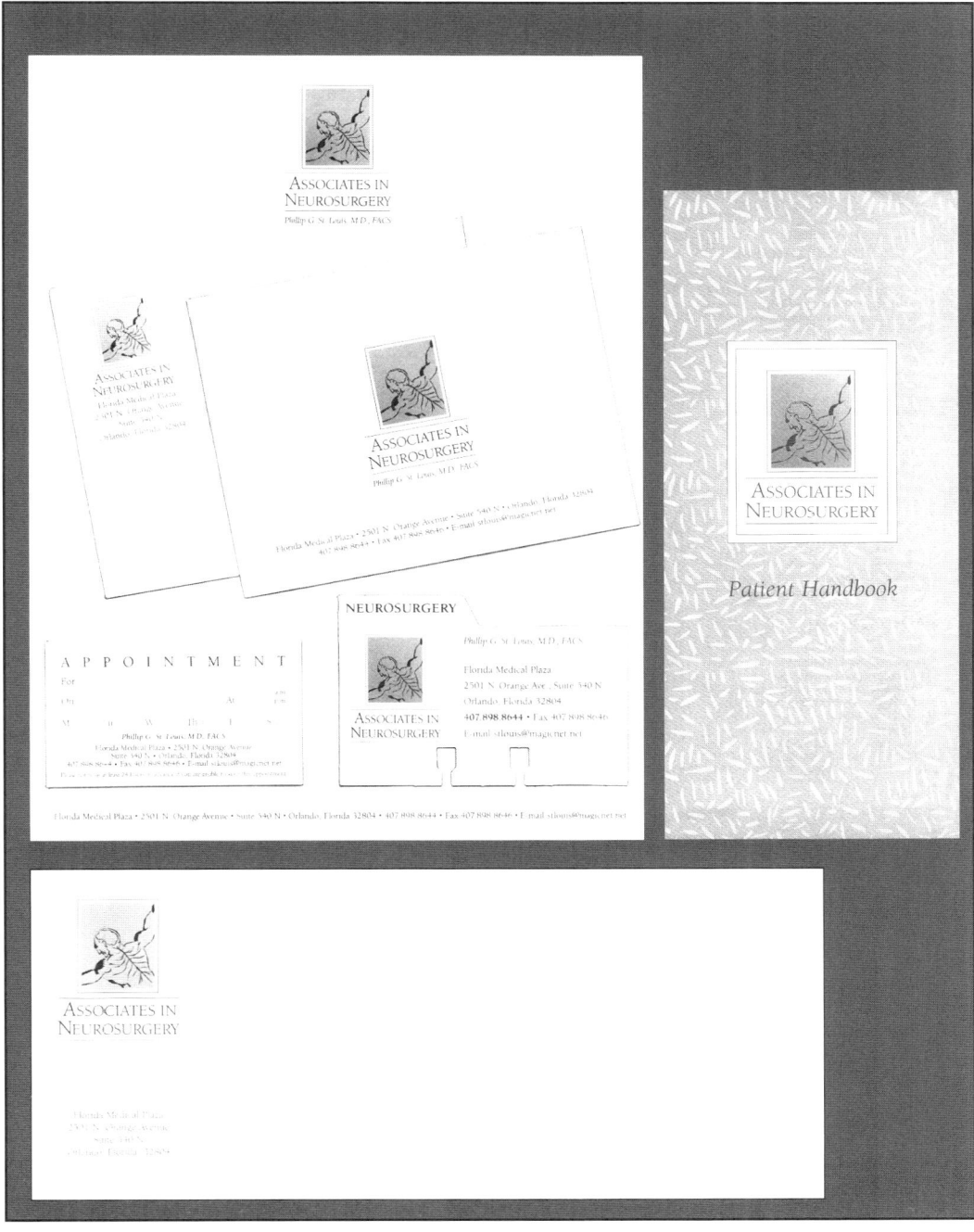

Cardiology newspaper ad

Working to keep you "heart healthy"

Since we began in 1979, we've been working to help Central Floridians live longer, healthier lives – to be "heart healthy." Along the way, we've grown to become one of the state's most dynamic leaders in the diagnosis, treatment and prevention of heart and blood vessel disease.

We evaluate and treat a variety of cardiovascular conditions and generally see patients for coronary artery disease (heart), peripheral artery disease (arms and legs) and arrhythmias (electrical problems of the heart). We also diagnose and treat chest pain, high cholesterol, high blood pressure, poor circulation, heart valve problems and heart failure.

All of our doctors are Board Certified or eligible for certification by the American Board of Internal Medicine in the subspecialty of Cardiovascular Disease.

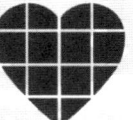

FLORIDA HEART GROUP, P.A.

Working to keep you "heart healthy"

615 East Princeton Street • Suite 300 • Orlando, Florida 32803 • 407-894-4474 or 1-800-28-HEART

Dermatology practice identity package

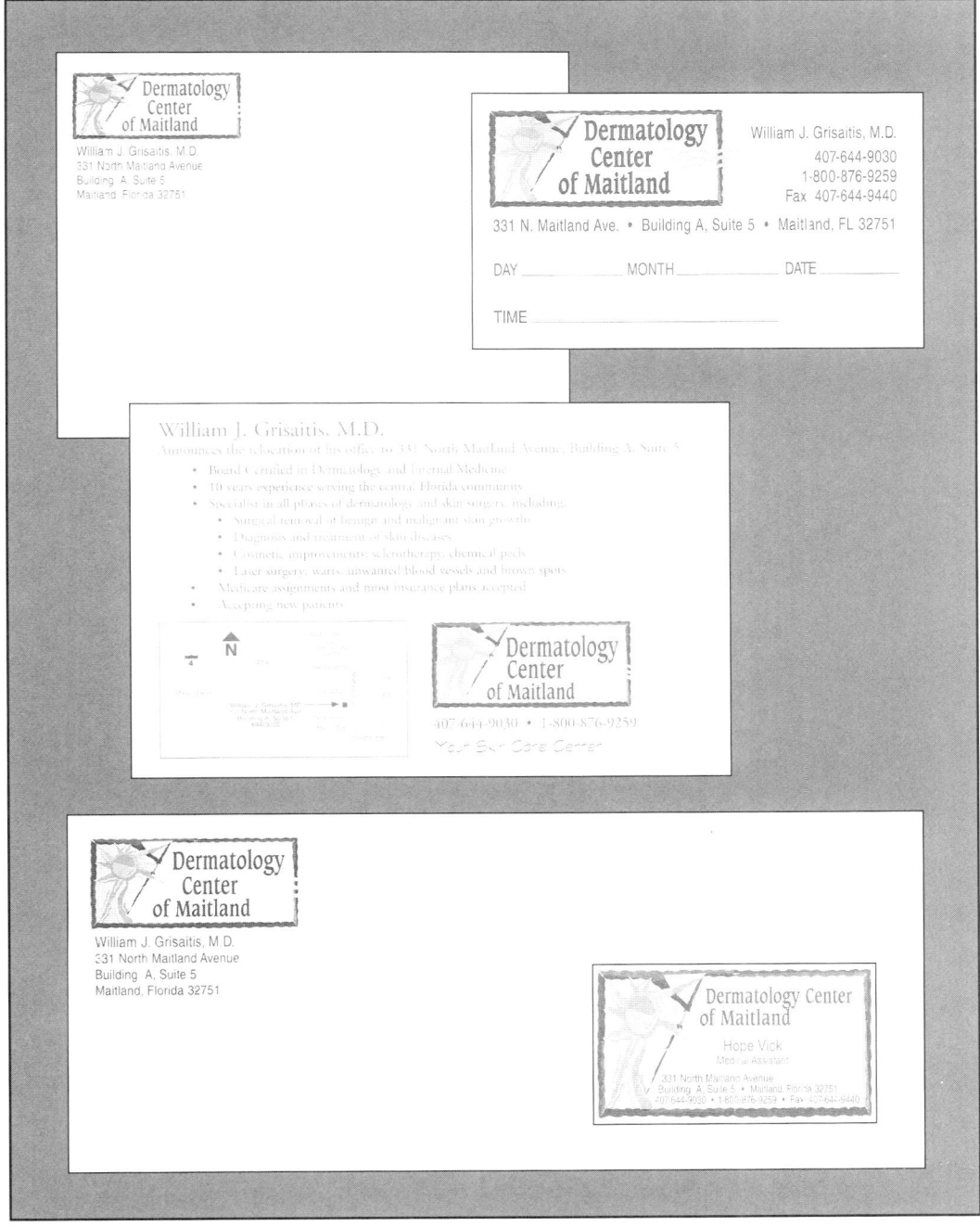

Practice services brochure

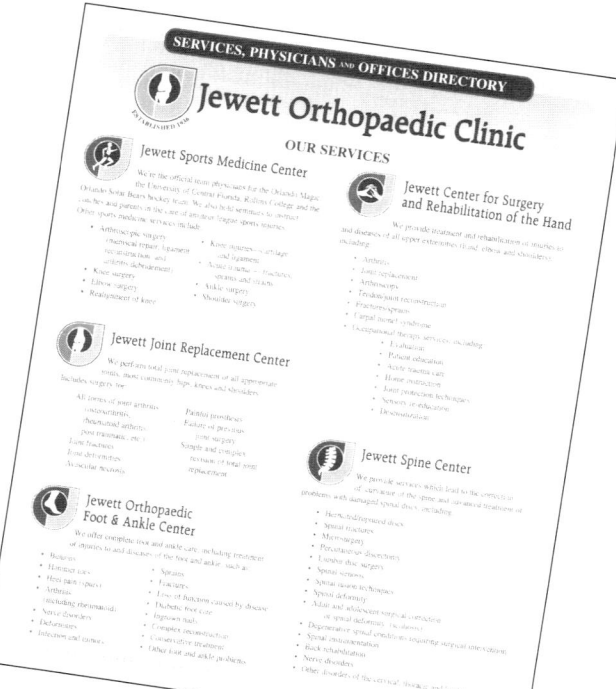

SERVICES, PHYSICIANS AND OFFICES DIRECTORY

Jewett Orthopaedic Clinic

OUR SERVICES

Jewett Sports Medicine Center

We're the official team physicians for the Orlando Magic, the University of Central Florida, Rollins College and the Orlando Solar Bears hockey team. We also hold seminars to instruct coaches and patients in the care of amateur league sports injuries. Other sports medicine services include:

- Arthroscopic surgery chemical repair, ligament recalculation and release/adjustment
- Knee surgery
- Elbow surgery
- Replacement of knee
- Knee injuries — cartilage and ligament
- Ankle trauma — fractures, sprains and sprains
- Ankle surgery
- Shoulder surgery

Jewett Center for Surgery and Rehabilitation of the Hand

We provide treatment and rehabilitation of injuries and diseases of all upper extremities (hand, elbow and shoulder), including:

- Arthritis
- Joint replacement
- Arthroscopy
- Tendon/joint reconstruction
- Fractures/sprains
- Carpal tunnel syndrome
- Occupational therapy services, including:
  - Evaluation
  - Patient education
  - Acute trauma care
  - Home instruction
  - Joint protection techniques
  - Sensory re-education
  - Demonstration

Jewett Joint Replacement Center

We perform total joint replacement of all appropriate joints, most commonly hips, knees and shoulders. Includes surgery for:

- All types of joint arthritis (osteoarthritis, rheumatoid arthritis, post-traumatic, etc.)
- Joint fractures
- Bone deformities
- Avascular necrosis
- Painful prosthesis
- Failure of previous joint surgery
- Simple and complex revision of total joint replacement

Jewett Orthopaedic Foot & Ankle Center

We offer complete foot and ankle care, including treatment of injuries to and disorders of the foot and ankle, such as:

- Bunions
- Hammer toes
- Heel pain (spurs)
- Arthritis (including rheumatoid)
- Nerve disorders
- Deformities
- Infection and tumors
- Sprains
- Fractures
- Loss of function caused by disease
- Diabetic foot care
- Ingrown nails
- Complex reconstruction
- Constructive treatment
- Other foot and ankle problems

Jewett Spine Center

We provide services which lead to the correction of disruption of the spine and elevated treatment of problems with damaged spinal discs, including:

- Herniated/ruptured discs
- Spinal fractures
- Microsurgery
- Percutaneous discectomy
- Lumbar disc surgery
- Spinal stenosis
- Spinal fusion techniques
- Spinal deformity
- Adult and adolescent surgical correction of spinal deformity (scoliosis)
- Degenerative spinal conditions requiring surgical intervention
- Spinal instrumentation
- Back rehabilitation
- Nerve disorders
- Other disorders of the cervical, thoracic and lumbar spine

OUR PHYSICIANS

James C. Barnett, M.D.
Arthroscopic and Reconstructive Surgery of the Knee

John W. McCutchen, M.D.
Hip Surgery

Gregory O. Munson, M.D.
Surgery of the Spine

John R. Chase, M.D.
Knee and Ankle Surgery

Richard L. Shure, M.D.
Hand/Microvascular Surgery

Hugh B. Morris, M.D.
Reconstructive Surgery of the Hip and Knee
Sports Medicine
Shoulder Surgery

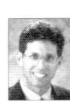
Richard M. Konsens, M.D.
Reconstructive Surgery of the Knee
Sports Medicine

Reginald L. Tall, M.D.
Surgery of the Spine

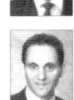
John A. Papa, M.D.
Foot and Ankle Surgery

Brian K. Barnard, M.D.
Hand/Microvascular Surgery
Arthroscopic/Reconstructive Surgery of the Shoulder

Janet M. Robison, M.D.
Arthroscopic and Reconstructive Surgery of the Knee
General Orthopaedics

Robert W. Westergan, M.D.
General Orthopaedics

Adam S. Fenichel, M.D.
Hand/Microvascular Surgery
Pediatric Orthopaedic Surgery

Joseph B. Billings, D.O.
Arthroscopic and Reconstructive Surgery of the Knee
Sports Medicine

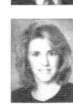
Colleen M. Zittel, M.D.
Rehabilitation Medicine and Electrodiagnosis

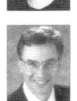
Wadih S. Macksoud, M.D.
Hand/Microvascular Surgery

Mary Lynn Brown, M.D.
Hand/Microvascular Surgery

Craig M. Mintzer, M.D.
Sports Medicine/Arthroscopic Surgery of the Shoulder and Knee
Pediatric Orthopaedic Surgery

Michael Mac Millan, M.D.
Surgery of the Spine

Steven A. Bohmer, M.D.
Arthroscopic and Reconstructive Surgery of the Hip, Knee and Shoulder

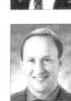
Kenneth A. Krumins, M.D.
General Orthopaedics
Arthroscopic and Reconstructive Surgery of the Knee
Sports Medicine

Mark A. Beckner, M.D.
Surgery of the Spine

Jeffrey A. Deren, M.D.
Hand/Microvascular Surgery

Specialty services brochure

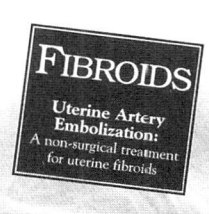

FIBROIDS

Uterine Artery Embolization:
A non-surgical treatment for uterine fibroids

Do you have fibroid tumors?
What do you do now?

- What are fibroids?
- What is Uterine Artery Embolization (UAE)?
- A real patient's story
- Why should I consider MCRG for my fibroid treatment?

MCRG
MEDICAL CENTER RADIOLOGY GROUP
Located at Orlando Regional Healthcare System
Fibroid Information: (407) 423-2581, ext. 244
This information is provided by the radiologists of Medical Center Radiology Group, specialists in diagnostic and interventional imaging, affiliated with the Orlando Regional Healthcare System.

Medical Center Radiology Group

is a multi-specialty radiology group practice located at Orlando Regional Healthcare System that brings state-of-the-art radiology services to Central Florida. MCRG has grown from a small practice in 1949 to 27 radiologists at six hospitals throughout the region. MCRG has had the confidence of Orlando's medical community for 50 years.

MCRG understands that its value comes in its role as an effective partner...with the patient who needs and deserves the most competent, caring health treatment available ... with the physicians who rely on MCRG professional services to complete their health care picture ... with the hospital that entrusts MCRG with its radiology needs ... and with the Central Florida community that it serves.

But MCRG is more than just a professional partnership. MCRG's real strength comes from the outstanding individuals in the practice. MCRG radiologists are among the most highly-trained and well-respected in their fields.

Among the skilled leaders on the Uterine Artery Embolization team:

Dr. Joseph G. Andriole, Chief of the Division of Interventional Radiology and Angiography at ORHS, is a Board-certified diagnostic radiologist with 15 years of experience. He has a special interest in the management of gynecological abnormalities. An expert in vascular and interventional radiology, his publications and presentations have received national recognition.

Dr. Joe F. Franklin is Board-certified in both diagnostic radiology and urology. He has extensive training in interventional radiology and angiography and has served as Chairman of the Department of Radiology at Orlando Regional Medical Center.

Medical Center Radiology Group Fibroid Information:
(407) 423-2581, ext. 244

H...

1. Call Medical Center Radio... at Orlando Regional Health... (407) 423-2581, ext. 244.
2. You will talk over the tele... Physician's Assistant at MCRG to... might be a candidate for UAE. Additional screening might include an UltraSound and an appointment with the radiologist.
3. UAE patients are admitted to Orlando Regional Medical Center for a "short stay", usually less than 24 hours.
4. An intravenous catheter will be started in your arm. Through that catheter, you will receive antibiotics and fluids.

...Lab for the ...cation for ...your catheter. ...ough a small ...h - in the groin ...es can be injected into the art... ...ff the blood flow to the fibroid.
7. Most patients are on bedrest for 4-6 hours following the procedure.
8. Many patients take medication for pain at home for several days afterward.
9. The fibroid tumor begins to shrink; even multiple fibroids shrink.

Uterine Artery Embolization

 terine Artery Embolization (UAE) is a relatively new procedure for the treatment of fibroids and their symptoms, so your regular doctor may not be familiar with it. Embolization is a well-established method for treating many types of bleeding, such as that in the uterus after childbirth. UAE is an innovative application of a proven technique.

UAE is based on the premise that fibroid tumors can be "starved out" by cutting off their blood supply. UAE is performed by an interventional radiologist, a physician who uses x-rays and other radiology tools to treat medical conditions without major surgery. The doctor uses sophisticated x-ray technology to find the artery that feeds the fibroids; then, he inserts tiny particles through a very small catheter into the artery, effectively blocking the fibroid's blood supply. The procedure is non-surgical; patients are hospitalized less than 24 hours and return to normal activity within a few days.

The idea is simple and the treatment is effective: 90% of patients experience significant relief from their pre-treatment symptoms.

UAE: A Real Life Story

 hirty seven-year-old Teresa, of Orlando, Florida, had abdominal pain so severe that she couldn't bend over to tie her own shoes. Her gynecologist found a fibroid tumor and his solution: have a hysterectomy.

Teresa was uncomfortable with major surgery to remove an organ that was otherwise healthy except for the fibroids, and she wasn't completely sure that she wouldn't want to have a child. It was the only option he could offer.

So Teresa did an Internet search for "fibroids" and discovered Uterine Artery Embolization. Her next gynecologist promptly referred her to Dr. Andriole at Medical Center Radiology Group at Orlando Regional Healthcare System in Orlando.

Utilizing ultrasound, Dr. Andriole found a second fibroid. He discussed various options with Teresa. She elected to have the UAE procedure. Six months later, ultrasound showed that her larger fibroid had shrunk by 75%, her second by almost as much, and her symptoms were completely gone. She feels "great!"

"My advice to women is 'learn as much as you can' and 'ask your doctor lots of questions'. The more you know, the better able you are to make the choice that's best for you."

Cardiology patient newsletter

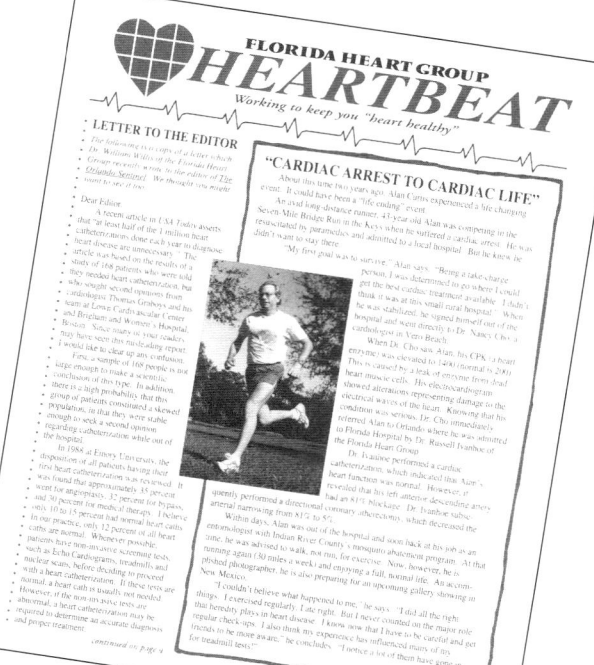

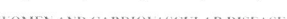

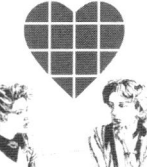

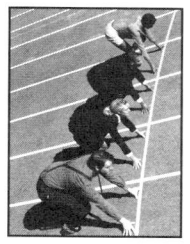

Resources

Blue, Barbara Ann, President, Business Performance Group, Inc., Tampa, Florida, 813-251-5010

Brandenburger, Adam M. and Barry J. Nalbuff, "The Right Game: Use Game Theory to Shape Strategy," *Harvard Business Review,* July-August, 1995, pgs. 57-71

Bruns, John F., General Manager, Ritz-Carlton, Cleveland, Ohio, 216-623-1300.

Cassidy, David, Marketing Director, Jewett Orthopaedic Clinic, Orlando, Florida, 407-647-2287.

Collis, David J. and Cynthia A. Montgomery, "Competing on Resources," *Harvard Business Review,* July-August 1995, pgs. 118-128.

Colvin, Geoffrey, "The Changing Art of Becoming Unbeatable," *Fortune,* November 24, 1997, pgs. 299-300

Frankel, Dan, Ph.D., Principal of Martin/Frankel Associates, 336-768-6466.

Gross, T. Scott, *Positively Outrageous Service,* Mastermedia Limited., New York. 1991.

Halbrooks, John R., ed., *How to Really Deliver Superior Customer Service,* Goldhirsh Group, Inc., Boston, Massachusetts. 1994

Hammer, Michael and Steven A. Stanton, "The Power of Reflection," *Fortune,* November 24, 1997, pgs. 291-296

Kim, W. Chan and Renee Mauborgne, "Value Innovation: The Strategic Logic of High Growth," *Harvard Business Review,* January – February 1997, pgs. 103-112

Kodzis, Bob, Founder, Flight of Ideas, Orlando, Florida, 407-699-7484.

Kriegel, Robert J. and Louis Patler, *If it ain't broke...BREAK IT!,* Warner Books, New York. 1991

Krohn, Richard, *Physician Networks, Strategy, Start-Up and Operation,* ACHE Management Series, Health Administration Press, 1998

LeBoeuf, Michael, Phd, *How to Win Customers and Keep Them for Life,* Berkley Books, New York. 1989

Nulman, Philip R., *Start Up Marketing,* Career Press, Franklin Lakes, New Jersey. 1996.

Peters, Tom, *The Pursuit of WOW!,* Vintage Books, New York. 1994

Schaaf, Dick and Ron Zemke, *Taking Care of Business,* Lakeland Books, Minneapolis, Mn. 1991

"Strategies for the Healthcare Marketplace," *The Alliance Report.* March 1999

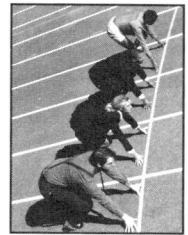

Index